ROSINA, THE MIDWIFE

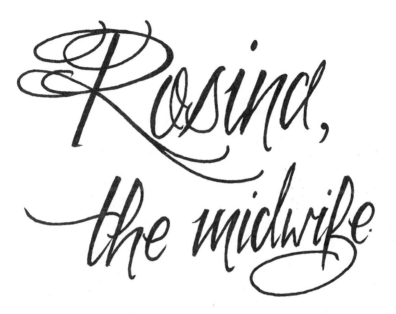

Rosina, the midwife

JESSICA KLUTHE

Tony,
I hope you enjoy
this story!
    Non basta una vita!
                J Kluthe

BRINDLE
& GLASS

Brindle & Glass Publishing Ltd.
brindleandglass.com

LIBRARY AND ARCHIVES CANADA CATALOGUING IN PUBLICATION
Kluthe, Jessica, 1985–
Rosina, the midwife / Jessica Kluthe.

Also issued in electronic format.
ISBN 978-1-927366-11-0

1. Russo, Rosina. 2. Midwives—Italy—Calabria—Biography. 3. Calabria (Italy)—
Biography. 4. Russo family. 5. Italian Canadians—Biography. I. Title.

DG975.C155K58 2013   618.2'0233092   C2012-906797-0

Editor: Linda Goyette
Proofreader: Heather Sangster, Strong Finish
Cover image: Henry Roxas
Tile texture: Michael Richert, RGBStock.com
Cover lettering, map, and family tree: Karl Sundquist
Design: Pete Kohut
Author photo: Billie Depatie, D4 Photography

Brindle & Glass is pleased to acknowledge the financial support for its publishing
program from the Government of Canada through the Canada Book Fund, Canada
Council for the Arts, and the Province of British Columbia through the British
Columbia Arts Council and the Book Publishing Tax Credit.

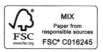

The interior pages of this book have been printed on 30% post-consumer
recycled paper, processed chlorine free, and printed with vegetable-based inks.

1 2 3 4 5 17 16 15 14 13

PRINTED IN CANADA

For you, Rosina Vecchia.

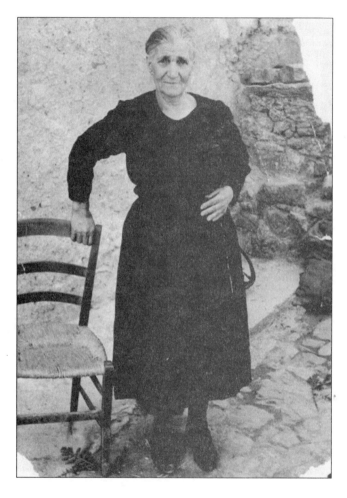

I find myself remembering dry ditches with sparse grasses. Sometimes, gravel on roadsides or damp mornings. Other times, a door frame or the persistence of a poppy. Sometimes, it's the shadows around her eyes.

CONTENTS

✤ ✤ ✤

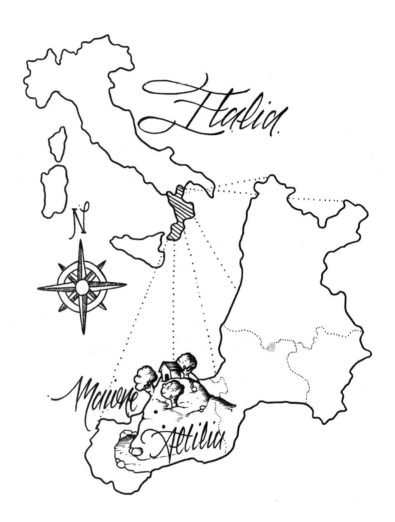

U N O

trace a light line left on a map to mark a traveller's
passage

*She dangles there. A sort of crucifix over my doorway. I don't have
much. A name—three syllables. Ro. Si. Na.*

*There is no song to help me feel her, no voice to remind me of hers.
There is no scent, no texture. No time of day.*

She died in 1969, sixteen years before I was born.

It was late fall the first time that I really saw her. Everything was
wet, rotting. Branches like raw knuckles. The Nanking cherries,
instead of letting go, held on tighter—solid black raisins for the
birds to peck. The crabapples exploded, burst and shrivelled far

below the once-bright sky, their skins deflated red balloons. As I ran up the front steps, my breath clung to the air, a blurry stream. I yanked open the door and knew that the furnace was on; I smelled lint and hair and whatever else had collected in the heat vents since spring.

I was in the basement digging out my winter clothes when I found her. I had hauled out all of the boxes and bins from under the stairs and tried to squeeze myself into my former hide-and-seek spots to look for the partner to a mitten. My parents' crawl space was a collection site for objects that didn't have year-round positions, relocated hall closet and junk drawer items like rubber boots and tobacco tins full of fence-board nails.

I found the photo inside a box that also held a *Company's Coming* cookbook, a brown velvet pincushion, and an oil lantern. The picture was a copy, enlarged from a smaller print, distorted in length. I blew off the dust and watched the tiny particles sway in the air before they found new surfaces to land on. And there she was—Rosina.

She is wearing a long dark dress, cinched in at the waist. Her hair, mostly white, is pulled back from her face. Deep circles surround her dark eyes. Her hands are wrinkled like crushed paper. With one hand she holds on to a wooden chair, the other rests on her hip. She stands there on worn stones, in front of an old stucco wall, almost smiling.

Only this one photo of her was ever taken, or at least that is what everyone says. Nanni Rose keeps a copy in a cabinet, between gold-rimmed teacups and the dishes that are never used. When she speaks of Rosina, she glances toward the cabinet. If we are sitting at her kitchen table, sipping thick espresso out of tiny cups, she will peer over my head at it. If we are in the backyard, she will look toward the house. On holidays, when Nanni pulls out the wine glasses or platters, she will pause there a moment before returning to the pots boiling on the stove. Sometimes she will say, "Come. Come. I will show you," but it is hard to get a clear view through the cabinet's crystal doors. She taps on the glass with her finger, and I peek in. Before asking me when I plan to have children, she always mentions that Rosina was an *ostetrica*, a midwife. She always nods before I answer. *She delivered hundreds. Hundreds.* It's always hundreds.

This was as close as I had ever been to Rosina. I took the photo out of the frame and turned it over to see if anyone had printed on the back. No year. No place name. Nothing but *Rosina vecchia*. Old Rosina.

I wondered what existed outside the frame. Another chair? Did the stucco wall belong to her house? Where did she live and with whom? Who stood behind the lens? I packed up the box, except for the oil lantern and the photo, and sat a while on the basement floor before filling in the hiding places with boxes and hauling my winter clothes upstairs. I played around with the lantern; it wasn't the kind you take camping. The glass was thin, and the handle wasn't made for function. It was probably bought at one of those estate auctions, along with that box of glass negatives, those slides of strangers who stare at us with piercing eyes, backwards, their clothing more visible than their faces. I stayed there, trying to light the lantern and imagine her. But the frayed wick would not catch long enough to make a steady flame.

❧ ❧ ❧

She runs, alive with the night, shocked that it is happening so soon. Shadows spread across a worn path. The bright moon flashes between the trees and collides with the glassy light of the lantern in her hand as she goes. Her shadow rushes over the bony silhouettes of the trees on either side, lost to the darkness, to be lit up again in a stride. She had thought she would have at least another two weeks, maybe three, but when her neighbour tapped on the door just as she started to fall asleep, she knew.

"I'll come with you," she offered.

"No. No. You stay here. Rest. It's late."

She knows the ground well, even in the dark. She slows down around the spots where rotting roots have left holes and takes wider strides over a nettle patch; her legs are bare beneath her gown. There's a rush that comes with a night birth. A baby slips in to the world while neighbours are asleep in darkened houses and wayward husbands slumber somewhere under the stars. Nearby female relatives—aunts, sisters, mothers, and cousins—are awake and alert, ready to assist the midwife, to welcome new life. The exhausted mother pleads for rest in the seconds between the contractions that attack her body, force it to twist into a knot around her belly. She spits out the name Gesù! and belts hard *ahhhs* from her throat after she swallows strings of vomit.

When a flickering light in the window comes into view, Rosina runs faster, snapping the brittle grass as each foot smacks the ground. She feels dizzy; the tall trees look like deep green smudges, but the stars stay in place. She concentrates on planning her movements, imagines what could happen. What she will do if there is too much blood. If the water has not broken. If the cord is tangled. If the baby is crowning, or if its legs are pushing through first. *She's done this hundreds of times. Hundreds.*

She plunges her hands into a pail of water on the porch, splashing moonlit water onto the wooden steps. As she yanks open the door, heat from the fireplace flashes against her cheeks. In the corner, coffee boils on the stove, preparation for the long night ahead. The scent of dark beans and blood curls in the air. In haste she lets her bag slump off her shoulders and fall to the floor. The bag is teeming with herbal remedies, homebrews in corked jars. Puffy aloe leaves, cabbage, and containers of clover. Cotton cloths, pressed and folded. Forceps, scissors, and sewing needles.

An oil lantern, hanging from a ceiling beam, spills pale yellow light across the floor. Women stare at her. They shuffle to make space and then look to her for direction. One says, "Come. Come. We've been waiting."

With her hands on the labouring woman's sticky thighs, her hip hard against the bed frame, Rosina presses the woman's legs apart and counts the number of beats between shudders. She instructs the others. You, hold her legs back—farther. And you, rub a damp cloth on her neck and lips to keep her cool. And someone, open the window and let the breeze in. Rosina's heart thumps deep in her chest and an ache throbs behind her eyes, making it impossible to keep track. The others count; she trusts their heavy whispers. The woman has been pushing already and is soaked in sweat, and shaking. Her hands, balled into tight fists, are white, and her veins, bright purple lines, are thick with blood. Rosina takes the mother's hands into her own. Damp skin sticks to her palms. She uncurls the woman's fists, reminds her to breathe, and with two fingers to the wrist feels her pulse. Rosina brushes away the black curls stuck to the woman's forehead and neck. She steps back for a moment and looks at the mother—two round breasts atop one round belly, swollen feet and fingers, puffy eyelids and lips, back arched, pushing everything she has forward. She is ready. The bed sheets are stained with bright blood. Some women speak to Mary. Some ask Mary to speak to God. *Let the surges stop. Let the baby come.*

After a night of labour—the entire house heaving together—a baby is born. Sunlight creeps in beneath the brown velvet curtains: a too bright, unwelcome rising. Daylight reveals lines of brown blood, tiny dry rivers, following the cracks of the floorboards. The women stare at the ground, following the rivers with their eyes, tracing the flow. The mother cries out to Mary, Mother of God, and a still infant never wakes to see the morning.

Rosina swaddles the tiny body in a thin white sheet, creasing the folds. After brushing eyelids closed, she pulls the top edge over the baby's blue face. She kisses the child's forehead and then crosses it with her fingertips. She rests the baby girl in her weeping mama's arms. Whispering gentle instructions, Rosina tells the woman to stay in bed for a least one week, to let her body pull back together. To eat a cupful of chicken broth and drink water, a teaspoon at a time. She peels off a cabbage leaf for the woman to tuck into her dress against her breasts to prevent cracking. First, she instructs, squeeze out the unneeded milk. She'll be back in a day or two to check in, to make sure there is no infection, no more bleeding.

Without letting her voice break, she whispers, "God bless," and then leaves the house. She puts her hands into her apron pockets and nods up at the bright morning sky as she follows the dusty path back home.

❧   ❧   ❧

Later I sat at the kitchen table and watched my older sister, Melissa, put in the filter. Measure out the grounds. She moved around the kitchen until the coffee had brewed. The women in my family could glide through the kitchen, from sink to cupboard, oven to stovetop. They could double or triple a recipe without missing an ingredient. They spoke in pounds and ounces, thyme and oregano. "Don't worry about it," they would say to me when I tried to help. "You'll just have to marry a man who can cook."

Once, we had a family reunion inside a wood-panelled community hall that smelled of cellar. Next to the table, among too many open bottles of Coke, were rows of lasagna in oven-wide silver pans. I guess no one had specified what to bring. The pans were filled with the same long, scalloped-edge noodles, sliced eggs, and globs of tomato sauce. Nanni snuck up behind me and, with her cheek against mine, whispered, "Pick the best one." I spotted hers right away. I had watched her make it dozens of times. Her final touch: fresh Parmesan shaken through the fingers.

Melissa had practically lived with Nanni—Rosina's granddaughter—for the first years of her life. Nanni and Nonno always tell the story of waiting in line all night at Toys "R" Us for the release of the Cabbage Patch dolls. Was it 1976? Or the next year? They elbowed young parents as they rushed through the doors to the big green display. The doll came with a birth certificate. Melissa was the first one of her friends to have one, and they were just as proud as she was.

"I didn't have dolls. I dressed up zucchinis," Nanni always finishes. "Cradled them in my arms. Tucked them in at night."

"Yep. Yep. So'd my sisters," Nonno always adds. "Zucchinis."

After the Toys "R" Us story, the table would grow quiet. Family members would move the food around on their plates, or inspect their cuticles. Mom would change the subject. Nanni and Nonno were the ones in line at the store because Mom had been too busy growing up; she had Melissa at seventeen with some man who wasn't my dad.

In a way, I was jealous. Melissa had been part of Nanni's inside world while spending entire days with her. She collected all of Nanni's secrets over pound cakes, and all the stories about Calabria—the Old Country—while picking peas or peeling apples. She watched Nanni brush her hair. Fold towels. Tie back the tomato plants with strips of old pantyhose. I was told watered-down, second-hand versions of stories, and only when I asked.

Melissa would tell me things like Nan didn't say yes to Nonno until they moved to Canada. That she was promised to another man, and he immigrated at the same time too. That the man lived in Edmonton and he sometimes went over there for dinner or for a barbecue. Nanni was still young when she took care of Melissa, and so her memories were still ripe.

I had gone over to my sister's house that afternoon to find out what she knew about Rosina, what Nanni had told her.

"I don't think I know much more about Rosina than you. When I opened the email I recognized the picture. Her slight smile. Reminds me of Nan. Glad you scanned it," Melissa said while pouring the coffee and pushing sugar cubes across the table. "I think I will print it out and frame it."

Something. Tell me something.

"You know, I used to spend every day with Nan, and she would tell me that she used to spend all of her days with Rosina. Even though Rosina was Nan's grandmother, she was like a mother to Nan. She was closer to her than anyone else," Melissa said.

I thought about the Cabbage Patch story, and the way Nanni treated Melissa like a daughter. I imagined Nanni tucking that yarn-headed, freckled doll into bed next to Melissa, so she could wake to find it. Wake to be a little mother.

"What else do you know about Rosina?" I asked.

"I can't really remember. When you're a kid, you don't really listen to all those stories, you think they will always be there. You can always ask to hear them again and again. Each time only remembering a few things."

I needed to know about Rosina because I sensed that somewhere inside my belly was a baby; I didn't yet have the kind of words I needed to tell anyone about it, or the courage to find out for sure. I needed her—matriarch, midwife, mother. And Melissa was my way into Rosina's world.

I had almost told Mom about my missed periods earlier that morning, but she would have been too practical. Before I was ready to know for sure, she would have made me find out. Find out if I needed to grow up too fast. Melissa, at twenty-nine, was almost like a second mother. She was someone I could go to with questions I didn't want to ask anyone else: how to kiss, how to get over a heartbreak, how to have sex. And now, I was nineteen, just two years older than Mom had been when she was carrying Melissa and I needed to know how to deal with this situation.

Melissa tapped her hand on the table. "I do remember one thing. Nan told me that she used to sleep in Rosina's bed with her, just like I used to sleep with Nan. Nan would kick Nonno out, and I would get to spend the night in their room. Nan used to sleep with Rosina, partly because their place was so small, but also because she wanted to. Nanni always wanted to be near her, like a little shadow."

I thought of Nanni's stories. She would wake up in the night when Rosina was preparing to leave for a delivery. Nanni would sit up on her knees, careful not to let the bed creak because she didn't want to wake anyone else. She would peek though the window, squinting into the night until her grandmother, delivery bag in hand, had disappeared into darkness. In the morning, she'd ask to hear all about the baby. And sometimes, in the days that followed, she would be allowed to go with Rosina to check on a new mother or to bathe a baby, check its skin colour and its little thump, thumping heart.

Melissa put her hand on her shoulder and pulled it forward, leaned her head back and looked up at the ceiling. I took the opportunity to really look at her—at the dark curls that fell over her shoulders, at her brown, deep-set eyes—we looked alike despite the ten years between us, and despite our different fathers. She didn't say anything for a while until, with her perfectly arched eyebrows scrunched together, she asked, "Why are you suddenly so curious about Rosina?"

I shrugged, then lied. "Just because I found her picture, I guess."

My sister let the silence move across the kitchen. I leaned toward the baker's rack piled with recipe books and pretended to be reading the titles on the spines. Eventually, she spoke of the only line that connected them. And now a line—however faint—that connected me.

"You know when you lose a baby more than once, they start to look into your family history."

"Oh yeah?" I responded, feeling myself flush. I reached for a recipe book, *Slow Cooker Meals*, and fanned through the pages.

"They didn't find out anything really," Melissa said. "I guess sometimes women just lose babies. For me that was the first time I really thought about her. You know, Rosina was a midwife and she gave birth five times just like Nanni and Mom. And here I was, losing baby after baby. I just thought about her. I don't know why. It's important to know about your history, at least the medical stuff."

My sister was looking right at me.

I stared down to watch my sugar cube dissolve. Pieces of the cube floated on the milky surface, then sank. I told her about the box with the lantern and velvet pincushion, told her the story about Rosina dashing through the night, the bony trees and open field.

"I think I've heard that story before."

"No. I wrote it after I found her picture. I imagined it."

"Are you sure? I think I've heard it before."

D U E

projections a system of lines that run parallel to
imaginary ones

Jenny swung open the curtain, rushing the hooks along the
U-shaped rail. Nothing was left between her and what the patient
had left behind—sometimes it was a snotty rag, sometimes it was
a chewed Styrofoam cup, sometimes it was an *Alberta Venture*
magazine with a curled top corner.

As always, she started with the bed. She clicked down the silver
handrail and shook the pillow out of its case. She heaved off the
blanket and this time found some crumpled panties. In one motion,
she stuffed the panties into the garbage, pulled the red plastic
drawstrings in opposite directions, and twisted them together into

a bow. The bag, not even half full, slumped to the floor.

She pulled off the sheets and reached for the fresh linens. With the clean blanket folded down at the top, she peeled her gloves down at the wrist and into themselves. Next, it was two pumps of blue disinfectant before bumping the cleaning cart out of the way. She wiped down the handrail and the arms of the chair. With her fingernail, she chipped at some gum on the wheel of the bed and then sprayed the disinfectant on the doctor's chair and desk. She leaned forward to wipe down the keyboard and computer screen. And there it was. Suspended in a small jar—just an inch from her face—backlit from the glow of the white screen a few inches behind it.

Two pinhead black eyes. A tiny pink curled body surrounded by a thick liquid. On the lid, it read: by-product of pregnancy.

"Room ready?" a nurse asked while she held up a man by his shoulders.

Jenny reached for the jar. She cupped it in both of her hands so that the patients in the corridor wouldn't see it and brought it over to the head nurse.

"You can discard that," she said.

"Sorry I took so long, but I had to change. I had a pretty messy night," Jenny told me as she slid into the car, pulling in with her the crisp rush of a winter night. Her scrubs were poking out the top of an IGA bag. She let the plastic bag crinkle to the floor.

"Messy? That's sort of disgusting," I said as I signalled the turn out of the hospital's parking lot toward the highway and prepared myself for the details. We waited at a red light, and when it changed—three bright green smudges on the icy windshield— Jenny pressed back into her seat.

She had been a volunteer in the ER for a few months, where she cleaned and prepared rooms; she hoped the job would help her decide if she wanted to go to nursing school. We were nothing alike when it came to gag reflexes. I couldn't even take out the garbage without my stomach turning, just another fact that encouraged the family comments about me needing to marry a good man.

When Jenny and I met in Grade 6, after my mostly friendless elementary school years, I knew I would be okay. By Grade 7, we refused to spend any time apart. At the beginning of the school year—after a summer of willing it to happen—we both got our first periods. In mock secrecy, girls passed each other tampons and pads, which we soon learned were a currency of womanhood. Girls rustled the plastic wrapping in the school bathroom, though I'm certain many unopened packages went straight into the garbage in the washroom stall.

That winter Jenny and I started to get our periods on the same day every month, a ritual that we later manufactured when we each started birth control. Every month we would lie on our beds, chewing on ice cubes with heating pads on our stomachs, complaining. Sometimes we were forced to complain over the phone or email, but either way the moment was shared— menstrual synchrony.

We practised other forms of sameness and often wore matching clothes. Once, on a field trip from Morinville, our small town, to a theatre in nearby Edmonton, the bus braked at a red light. To the right of the bus two young girls walked across a schoolyard, wearing matching shirts, pants, and sandals. Rob, the loudest guy in our class, yelled, "Hey, look!" while pointing at the girls. Everyone turned. "It's mini matching Jenn and Jess!" he exclaimed. The entire class started to laugh, and we slumped down into the vinyl seat, exchanging slight smiles. When we got a little older, we stopped matching but still coordinated colours and styles; other than our clothing we really looked nothing alike.

Jenny, taller than me with long blond hair and green eyes, tended to flaunt her Dutch heritage. She'd eat salty licorice candies and demonstrate her knowledge about Amsterdam though she'd never been to the city. *Did you know Van Gogh lived in Amsterdam? Well, he did.* I was a little shorter with dark curly hair and dark eyes and couldn't even try to pass as Dutch. When some of our friends started calling me "Ferrari" after they discovered my mother's maiden name, I was happy to take on this identity. I decided to live up to my new nickname by bringing Italian pastries to school, dipping biscotti into my hot chocolate, and putting Italian labels on things to learn the names. *La porta. Il libro. L'orologio.*

Regardless of our physical differences, people used our names interchangeably—Jessy to Jenny and Jenny to Jessy—and we rarely corrected anyone. We practised mimicking each other's printing until eventually, after some compromises on the curl of certain letters, we developed one indistinguishable style.

We filled notebooks for six years until our language became so alike that it seemed unnecessary to go on. Who was who? Years came to be represented by certain collections of notebooks and spoke for time in pages filled: the green leather book to black book time, the summer after that floral book that didn't have any lines.

The year after high school, we closed our notebooks and stopped writing to each other altogether, but we found other ways to connect. We managed to live through each other, blurring borders. She could recite Wilde's poetry after my university course on Late Victorian Literature. On days off work, she would come to my lectures. I could smell her baby-powder palms after she wore the rubber gloves and I knew the names of the hospital instruments and exactly what was in the drawers of the cleaning cart, like the paper-wrapped tongue depressors and orange urine sample containers. She read my notes and books and edited my papers. And I let her feel my bones and muscles to help her memorize the body.

Sometimes, I think it may be possible to live more than one life at a time, or at least imagine another life so fully it feels real, feels lived—life synchrony.

※   ※   ※

On my way to pick up Jenny after her shift, I'd imagine what she would be doing in the hospital, a place I could only enter upon complete necessity. When Melissa was giving birth to her first baby, my first niece, I forced myself to visit to offer support and share in the joy. While sitting in the waiting room, I would glance over at the closed venetian blinds on the long rectangular window beside the door to her room. I'd watched the white-robed doctors bump in and out of the doors down the hall. They were accessorized with stethoscopes, blue masks, and white-card key passes that I imagined permitted them to enter the bowels of the hospital, the places where no lost patient, scooting to the washroom or waiting room, would want to wander. Sometimes a nurse in scrubs and white running shoes would squeak to a stop near the delivery room door to read the chart documenting what was going on behind those sterile walls. I'm sure that the chart listed standard medical details: heart rate, age, weight, blood type, allergies. Somewhere on the chart, I assume, it mentioned Melissa's miscarriages. But it was missing footnotes about how scared she was carrying this baby and how she cried in Mom's arms and said that she just needed to take a hot bath and to keep something down.

When Melissa cried out, I looked over at those plastic ivory strips and imagined what was going on between those millimetre spaces. Mom was with her, I could hear her determined voice in the moments between contractions, and soon Melissa would be part of some female experience that I couldn't even witness. Afterwards, I understood her membership in the way that Mom looked at her: long blinks, slight nods. They had shared in something.

When I finally did go into her room—after the delivery was over—I saw metal tools resting in the sink and a turquoise bean-shaped pan dotted with spots of bright blood. My knees were weak as I walked over to my sister. I gripped the handrail of her bed for support and peeked at the sleeping baby girl in her arms. The moment I looked into that round face, my niece Hannah, wrapped and safety-pinned in a soft white receiving blanket, I was certain of the existence of God, of the Virgin Mother. And when Hannah wailed, a full-voiced scream from her belly, I felt a tug, some celestial certainty, which I hadn't felt in my body before. I'm not sure what made me faint: perhaps the swells of love rising up in me, or the IV poked into my sister's hand, or the clear tube up the side of her arm, or the peripheral of medical supplies, gauze, wires, and machines that flashed and buzzed. But the edges of the room went black just as soon as I realized my legs were softening beneath me. I'm sure if it had been Jenny's sister, she would have burst into the room with a bouquet of flowers. No staring at the blinds. No memory of the bean-shaped pan. No darkness at the edges.

That night, as we drove down the highway, Jenny spoke in a whisper. She did not tell her story to make me squirm or to cause my toes to curl. She said it bent forward, toward me. I pulled over. Two long beams of light, shining through thick white flakes, guided us to the shoulder.

"Pinhead eyes? You had to hold the jar?"

"Yeah. When I picked it up, it was warm."

The dim green dashboard light left her face in shadow. She reclined her seat. She was waiting for me to say something, but I didn't know how.

"It's okay," she finally said.

I tilted my head and looked at the roof.

"Jess, I know you've missed a couple periods," she said.

I had already felt the deep beat that muffled other people's words, pulsed in place of vowels. That deep beat had forced me to imagine the future every time he looked at me with those blue, bright eyes. I knew, when I told him, that he'd pull me close, rest his chin on the top of my head, and sling his arms around my shoulders. I knew he would think it would be okay. We'd have to stay in the town of seven thousand people whose faces we had seen a million times. Would we live with one set of parents? Maybe we could live with his parents, if they didn't hate me for this? I worked in a two-metre-by-two-metre gas bar; he worked outside even in the harsh Alberta winter so that we could afford to go on a trip to Italy, even though he would rather be creating art. We aimed to get out of there. Try on different lives. And now we'd be in this town forever without even knowing where else there was to go.

I followed the crack in the windshield from one side to the other. I would be with *this* man, my first boyfriend, my first love, and I would live in *this* town and be a mother to *this* baby. And *this* is where my life separated from Jenny's. *This* is where my belly would grow while her periods kept coming. *This* is what would separate adolescence from adulthood. By the time I settled my gaze on a rock chip, circled around its nearly perfect contour, and tried to imagine how I would tell him, and then how I would tell my parents, Jenny gasped.

"But it was just suspended in there, Jessy. Not floating. But not sinking either."

"I'm sorry."

I leaned forward and hugged the steering wheel to my chest and pressed my forehead against the top of the cold windshield. We peeked up. Up at the tiny pinheads of light.

T R E

cartogram an altered map where a desired value
replaces land, area, or distance

When I was a child, I'd colour between the black borders of
continents and lakes. I'd snake my blue Laurentian pencil
crayon over rivers and I'd make brown triangles where there
were mountains. From my desk in Morinville, I could draw my
province in only a few seconds: the rectangle with the jagged
left corner. I'd find my town—a black dot—somewhere near the
middle. I'd always colour in the oceans with my pencil crayon
pressed firm against the page. The oceans were important,
bigger than all the land masses put together, and I knew that
they separated things.

These maps became my way of viewing elsewhere. When I'd imagine a foreign place, maybe Portugal, or Russia, or Thailand, I'd imagine it as one big shape. I did so even though I learned that millions of people lived in separate cities, and that thinner borders existed inside a country's thick black outline. When I imagined Italy, from my home on the other side of the Peacock Blue Atlantic, it was just one long landscape inside a thin boot.

It was easy to remember where our family was from, where Calabria was located: the very toe of the boot. Calabria ended just in the arch of the foot where it collided with Basilicata and the base of the ankle where it ran into Campania. I knew that in this foot-shaped region were three farming villages—Maione, Altilia, and Grimaldi. Rosina, the midwife, her husband, Giovanni, the farmer, and their five children lived in these places. Stories became a magnifying glass: a way to zoom in, rush through the black dot, and explode into a view of trails and trees, rivers and roads.

Stories would thrust me through these worlds—indistinct backdrops—a blur of grass, wheat, water, and sand, areas that the characters moved through, worked, walked. As I grew older, the stories became more detailed. The storyteller—Nanni, Nonno, Mom, an aunt or uncle—would slow down. Stop. Certain places would come into full view: a small stone house on a hill. A rushing segment of a river. A line of bold oak trees.

A tall wheat field high up on a steep hill. The places where characters spoke, slept, died.

❧   ❧   ❧

I can see Rosina's husband, Giovanni, fall forward and snap the wheat beneath his body, bend and break the brittle stalks. And I can imagine that in 1915, Rosina nursed eleven-month-old Generoso while her four daughters picked acorns off the oaks. She saw the evening turn bright orange—that hazy colour that hangs in the air before it dissolves into dark. She watched the girls through the small window. They were twisting nuts from the shells; their black curly hair, backlit by sunset, looked nearly red. Their laughter moved through the light, wrapped around Rosina.

Rosina rubbed small circles into her baby boy's back. She wondered when her husband would return. *Hail Mary. Full of grace. The Lord is with Thee.* He had already missed dinner. She saved him some sliced potatoes and watery beef soup. *Blessed art Thou among women. And blessed is the fruit of Thy womb.* He had left early that morning, before anyone else was awake. She heard the metal latch slide into the wooden notch: a thud that signalled morning. *Jesus. Holy Mary. Mother of God.* She convinced herself that he was just too busy to stop and come in. *Pray for us. Sinners. Now and at the hour. The hour.* He spent long hours in the field at this time of year. *The hour of our death.* Rosina studied baby Generoso's small, creased knuckles and tiny, moon-shaped nails until it grew too dark to see. She lit the candles, put sleeping Generoso on the bed, and waved her daughters inside. After eating bowls of boiled acorns, the girls went to sleep.

The door creaked as Rosina slipped outside. She stood to make sure her exit hadn't disturbed her sleeping children and then she ran into the field and pushed into the waist-high wheat. The stalks poked and scratched her legs beneath her long dress, but she kept running. Her head was spinning. She thought she would faint from dizziness. The tops of the wheat looked like they were swaying back and forth, a golden wave, but she forced herself to keep going.

And then she saw the black bottom of his shoes, toes to the ground, and she stopped. All her breath burst from her lungs, throat, mouth and into the air. She saw his wide frame flat against the ground and fell toward him. His cheek pressed against the clumpy soil. She collapsed on top of him, her face on his back and cried. She shook him by the shoulders. "Caro Dio!" she yelled. His body was heavy and limp. In the dark, she couldn't make out his features. His lips tasted of dust.

In the weeks before Giovanni died, he and Rosina had walked from Maione—one tiny dot—to Grimaldi—a slightly larger dot—an hour's stroll between walls of silvery olive trees. For them, this was a well-mapped route as they had often hauled crates of vegetables to sell at the market in Grimaldi. But on this trip, they were going to see Dr. Iachetta. I'm certain Rosina remembered the details of the visit, and likely replayed them once it was too late. When they arrived at his clinic, they banged the cast-iron knocker and waited in the shade of the cement archway over the doctor's step. The door, heavy on its hinges, groaned open, and Dr. Iachetta, in a buttoned-down, collared shirt, emerged into the bright street. He shielded his eyes with one hand and reached for Giovanni's hand with the other. Dr. Iachetta ushered them in to his clinic, the front room of his house. Giovanni's hat trembled in his hand. He pulled out a chair and dropped it to his lap. Rosina watched her husband— the veins of his thick arms bulged in the heat—he tugged at his shirt and twisted back into the chair. He had cleaned under his square nails with the tip of a knife the night before, and now, with clean hands, rolled the tip of his hat between his thumb and forefinger. She waited until Giovanni explained that he had come for a checkup before she leaned in to kiss the doctor on the cheeks and give him the loaf of bread she had made. Rosina knew Dr. Iachetta well.

Years earlier, the doctor had arrived at a home in Maione where Rosina was delivering a baby. Though she didn't have formal medical training, he witnessed her abilities. He knew of the many women whom Rosina had assisted as a midwife, a practice common in isolated villages. That night, he offered her a bag of birthing tools: his forceps and other prying tools, scissors to cut the umbilical cord, a bar of soap to clean her hands and arms, and some ointment for numbing the skin.

Dr. Iachetta depended on her. When he couldn't be with a patient in childbirth, she delivered the babies for him, based on her own birth experiences, the memory of the surges and swells of her own labours, and the experiences of helping women in her immediate family. She had learned to read patterns like the consistency of blood and the strength of the heart. She recognized moments that signalled the various stages of delivery, when it was time to bear down, how hard the stomach should be, how to press to find the legs and butt and head, and how far up she should find the baby inside the mother. She had watched births as a little girl while her mother and aunts helped other women; sometimes she peered from the doorway and sometimes she just heard the cries of labour pains from outside the house. She had seen her mother scrub blood out of bed sheets at the river and then boil them. Women in the villages had come to depend on Rosina's experience and her ability.

The village priest also depended on her. He couldn't always be there to bless babies, to say their first rites, or sometimes their last ones, and he, too, supplied Rosina with some tools: a bottle of holy water and a rosary to take with her on deliveries. This kind of agreement between doctors, priests, and midwives was longstanding and common. All the way back to the Council of Trent in 1546, nearly four centuries earlier, the Catholic Church had set out the rules: midwives were permitted to baptize babies, provide expertise in matters of women's health—instruct them on ways to prevent infection, the foods to eat, and how to breastfeed—and also bear legal witness, when called upon, for cases of illegitimate infants. Midwives, with these responsibilities, were respected members of the village, especially among other women.

From a chair in the corner of the room, Rosina watched as Dr. Iachetta adjusted the stethoscope and then slipped it under Giovanni's shirt and against his chest. She watched as the doctor listened to the thumping of Giovanni's heart. She'd felt the pulse in so many women's wrists and sometimes two fingers below the earlobe—she knew a healthy rhythm. Dr. Iachetta nodded, adjusted the stethoscope, and then nodded again. He listed terms he had no doubt learned in medical school but then explained that Giovanni's heartbeat was irregular. It was unstable. Even though Giovanni was only forty-six, he would have to quit farming, the doctor explained, because the physical labour was too demanding on his heart. Giovanni brushed the hair off his forehead and dropped his hat onto his head. He inspected his clean nails. Rosina had feared this diagnosis—Giovanni's chest pains and shortness of breath, she had thought, signalled a grave illness.

The next morning, Giovanni had stepped outside and pulled the door's metal handle, latch to notch. He had no other training than farming, and besides, other jobs were scarce, he told Rosina. Some of his cousins had gone to America for work; they said they were coming back once they had made enough money, but did she see any of them again?

All around them, on the neighbouring farms, they knew that inside the tiny farmhouses, people sat around the table, just like them, with little to eat. After their crops of olives had been delivered to landowners in the villages, peasants were left with the chestnuts and acorns shaken from treetops—boiled and tasteless.

Giovanni knew struggle first-hand. He had been born at the end of the 1860s, the decade that had seen the unification of Italy. Unification suggests pulling together; it is easy to imagine thatched sections of land stitched together with little brown Xs or plump regional borders dissolving into thin lines. Giovanni was raised in the shadow of this unification amid promises of land reform that would lessen human struggle in the south. His parents had dreamed of teeming baskets and cupboards too full to close. The population of Italy nearly doubled in size through the nineteenth century, and the agrarian south suffered under this weight. Unification seemed to offer a way forward. Yet as time passed, the land was divided into ever-smaller strips, and reduced acres for sharecroppers meant reduced wages.

Giovanni grew up on a farm that actually suffered after unification; the promises to his parents had never been fulfilled. The new industrial policy benefited the northern cities. Increased taxes exhausted small southern farmers who could only rely on their prayers for abundance. Peasants lacked power—only two percent of Italians had the right to vote, and that two percent owned property and had the benefit of an education. The First World War would temporarily keep people in their home countries, but it was no wonder that older cousins of Rosina and Giovanni, and some neighbours, saw the promise of wages in foreign countries, triple what they were in Italy, as an appealing option.

Despite her concern for her husband's health, Rosina knew that as a farm labourer, Giovanni's efforts in the field allowed him only fifty percent of the profits. The couple needed the little money that he earned and the vegetables he produced to barter for salt and flour. They had five children at home, and baby Generoso hadn't even had his first birthday. Rosina knew that her husband's sickness was beyond anything she could care for with cotton rags, breathing techniques, suction, and the right amount of force. No amount of aloe or cabbage or clover, no homebrews to draw out fever or herbal ointments to numb aches in the joints, could cure his overworked heart. She prayed that her husband would recover, that at age thirty-two, and with five children, she wouldn't have to spend the rest of her life alone. She asked Mary to watch over them, Her children, to keep them in good health. As a part of the rhythm of her day, while Rosina cooked, cleaned, gardened, and nursed, she sent prayers to the Holy Mother: *O Blessed Mary, Mary, Mother of God. Mary, Mary, mend my husband's heart.*

Giovanni was buried in the only cemetery in Maione. His gravestone should have read "Giovanni Russo: 1869–1915," but the family couldn't afford a stone grave marker. Instead, his last name was burned into a wooden cross. In twenty-five years, Rosina would have to pay to keep Giovanni in his plot; otherwise, as there was no space left for the dead, he would be taken out of his wooden coffin and his bones would be put into a ten-by-ten-inch box. That box would be placed into a communal tomb, and she would have nowhere to go rest and talk to her husband. In these difficult years immediately following his death, the First World War broke out and conditions became worse than even Giovanni could have imagined. Rosina simply couldn't afford to keep his bones in place. Nor could she afford to let her own broken heart slow her down.

❧ ❧ ❧

Between the boot-shaped borders, a box of Giovanni's bones lies buried. I know that the box is in a tomb with others' bones, somewhere in a hillside *cimitero*, as Nonno would call it. I remember being told that the name Calabria, a word that always sounded to me, as a child, like a sunset sound—a bright orange rising—meant fertile land. Long before I learned about the history and the struggle over this land that eventually forced many people to migrate in search of another way to make a living, this definition made sense to me. Fertile land. Giovanni had been a farmer. Rosina had given birth to five babies and delivered hundreds of others. On those maps I'd colour at my desk, the compass in the bottom corner reminded me that the sun would rise over the Tyrrhenian and sink over the Ionian Sea, creating ripples of Peacock Blue and Canary Yellow. It was easy to imagine Rosina, who didn't migrate like the rest of her family, and who lived long after Giovanni died, as a character in every Calabrian story. Drawn from traces of stories, these were my maps.

QUATTRO

meridian an imaginary connecting line from
north to south along a given string of points

I unfold stories of her. Ro. Si. Na. By the mid-1930s, she was a
young grandmother. I can imagine her on her way home after
the delivery of that stillborn baby. She plans to return to visit
the mother, to ensure she is taking steps to prevent infection and
check that she has pulled herself out of bed. Rosina is making her
way to the tiny house on the hill in Maione where she lives now
with her grown son Generoso and his wife, Michelina. The sun
hovers near the horizon. The day promises to be thick with heat.
She shields her eyes from the glare—*Buongiorno, Calabria.*

I pile them together, story over story. RoSiNa. She is exhausted and dizzy—the small rocks on the pathway look like they are rolling back and forth. She stops to focus her eyes on a branch bent over the path ahead. No animals have passed yet, and there's only one car in the area to whip up the dust, to stir the stones. That vehicle left yesterday afternoon and won't return from Grimaldi until sometime this evening.

Once, the driver, the son of one of her cousins, offered her a ride between towns while she was on her way to turn a breech baby, to slowly, slowly work the belly like dough. He had been transporting the mail and taking a passenger to see Dr. Iachetta. The driver had said it would be no problem, and she was grateful for the offer, but she knew she would get too dizzy if she sat down in the car. She felt like she was going to fall down just watching the tires turn as the car sped away. The car spun the dust up in thick circles, expelling a trail of white exhaust that became thinner and thinner as it headed toward Grimaldi.

She imagines herself crouching down but worries what her neighbours will think if they see her resting at the most productive time of day, the hours before the sun makes things slow down, the grass bend, the vegetables soft. She imagines stepping into the trees, under their leafy canopy, and resting, but she keeps walking. She is even more worried about how she would explain herself to Mussolini's men, or the men who worked for Mussolini's men, if they stopped her. It was still a shock to see outsiders. Their little white, worn villages rarely saw anyone from the cities, and if they did, it was someone's relative, come to stay for a while. If the men spotted her walking idly, they would question her; they would demand proof of who she was and where she lived. *Rosina Russo. Mother of Generoso.* Women should be at home, working on their farms, working in their houses. *We live there. That house, see?* And where was she coming from? *A delivery.* And where was her husband? *Long dead. He died in that the field, just over there.*

I stitch stories, threading together time. Ro-si-na. Just a few weeks earlier, the uniformed men had entered some of her neighbours' houses. Village residents whispered the words *Fascista, Fascismo,* and *Fascio* across the river, through open windows and in the fields while pressing a shovel into the dirt with the arch of a booted foot. The uniformed men didn't bother climbing the hill to approach her house; perhaps it was the steep slope that had spared them. Maybe they were attempting to approach from the north side, which would require the men to cross the river. Rocks and fallen tree trunks—put in place—provided a way to cross without getting wet to the thighs, but it was difficult for newcomers to navigate. Even though the men never made it to the house, their presence in the region was a reminder that this little stitch of land was a part of the Italian nation, not just of the village community. A vast country existed beyond Calabria's borders, ruled by the fist and grimace of Benito Mussolini after 1922. Even so, Rosina was governed, foremost, by God.

Elsewhere in Italy, the situation was tense for midwives. For those women even suspected of performing abortions there were consequences: lack of proof of this criminal activity was viewed as evidence of midwives' slyness. Midwives and doctors suspected of slowing the growth of the Italian race, a necessary component for Mussolini's push for a strong military and huge territory, came under surveillance. Abortion was punishable, but the Fascists' desire to identify anyone who stood in the way of national growth sparked a campaign to charge doctors and midwives for criminal acts, committed or not, to serve as warning. Even cases that had been long closed were reopened in a quest to convict. Midwives provided valuable services, especially to working-class women in their communities. While some local people were hostile toward midwives they viewed as immoral, others would come to their defence. People who offered midwives support were treated as accomplices.

In larger towns, complicit civilians set up stations, and people were expected to contribute whatever copper and gold they had because Italy's future depended on it. Long lists were made of the items people dropped off. The value of the goods was estimated and scratched down into a book. As the Fascist state became a belligerent force in Abyssinia and Europe, its citizens were told that after the war, they would get replacements. Replacement wedding rings. Replacement heirlooms. Rosina didn't know how she would cook for her son Generoso and his family if the men took her only pot. How could she boil the potatoes? Sometimes the men said they would bring aluminum replacements, but they rarely ever came back. Copper for bullets. Bullets instead of food.

Rosina only ate what she needed to be able to move, to take care of her grandson, baby Giovanni, and manage the household while Generoso and his wife, Michelina, worked. Michelina once declared that she never saw Rosina eat. She never saw her chew or swallow. Rosina told her not to worry and that she had everything she needed. Rosina's stomach usually burned, and the dizziness she always felt—a fuzziness in her head when she moved too quickly or sat up too fast—became even worse when she was hungry. Sometimes, if she went long enough without food, the burning stopped and she didn't feel anything.

Many neighbours had planned to go to the cities to find work, but after Mussolini came to power, most people stayed put. There had been talk that a new city, right there in the south, would be erected and would put them on the map: Mussolinia.

Generoso told Rosina about a man in Altilia who refused to give Mussolini's men his pots. Generoso had heard this story from another man when he was in Grimaldi selling tomatoes, and the story spread among the three villages. The Fascists pointed their guns at the man's head. The man's wife begged him just to be quiet, to let the men take what they wanted. They didn't shoot him, but they could have killed him, right there; he would have been slumped over the woodstove. In some versions of the story, he was dead on the mud floor of the kitchen, and his wife had to move in with her brother-in-law. Other stories made their way south from the cities. In Rome, in the courtyard of Fort Bravetta, two anti-Fascist men charged with the attempted assassination of Il Duce were chained to chairs. While seated, they were shot in the back.

In response to these stories, Rosina told Generoso that if the men came, he was just to give them what they wanted, anything at all. Stay out of politics, she said. She was afraid Generoso would resist, that he would end up dead on their mud floor, that she would lose her only son to heaven, where he would be with his father, her husband. Giovanni. Generoso. And God.

The church bells sound. It is already 9:00 AM. She fears that the bells will be next to go, to be melted down and reshaped, from worship to war, from bells to ammunition. She wipes her rough hands on her apron, and then stretches out her fingers to press out the lines. She rubs her thumbs back and forth into her palms, into the lifelines, and wonders if she could have done something more. Could have made that baby's heart beat. But then, God has a plan. But the infant never cried. Never parted its lips. The bells ring again, and the chiming smoothes into echoes.

She takes the long way home so that she can approach the

house from the back, stop in the field and collect herself before anyone in the family sees her. Before her daughter-in-law asks about the delivery, the baby's mother, and the baby. Before the younger woman can look at the floor, nod, say something about God. Surely, everyone would be awake, feeding the animals, pulling potatoes, and collecting eggs—if there were any.

Rosina stops beside the tallest oak, her favourite spot to collect acorns because the branches reach into one another. She sits down. The field is bent up in places and sunk down in others. As her fingers bump over the tree's knots, she imagines its rigid roots below the ground. In some spots, only small bits of the roots reach the surface and look like bones to be unearthed, nearly stone. She thinks that this tree must be older than time, somehow eternal. The blood on her dirty apron can never be completely washed out, even if she spends hours bent at the river. She tugs it off and ties the strings into a bow. She lets the linen crumble to the ground. She tries to stand up and leave, but something pulls her down, that deep beat, as resounding as the church bells. With her face in her hands, she lets her chest heave. She allows her tears to stream without making a sound.

That night, while Generoso and Michelina sleep, Rosina cradles her grandson, baby Giovanni. As she rocks him, hums into his ear as he tries to fight sleep, she wonders if this is her rightful job. To tug into the world, and to cradle. To bless these little loves so they can enter heaven. To carry them to christenings, and hold them before the Church as the one who pulled them into this world. She sings *al-le-lu-ia* to the sleeping baby on her shoulder as she imagines the other babies who will be born between those stone walls. She prays that they'll come into the house hollering, and with fists in the air. *Al-le-luuu-ia. Al-le-e-luuu-ia. Amen.*

In this house on the hill, a baby girl is born next, a blessing that arrives a few weeks before Christmas 1938. Rosina swaddled her red-faced grandbaby, not yet a minute old, and placed her in Michelina's arms. "Amen," Rosina said before she yelled out the window for Generoso. He burst into the room with Giovanni toddling underfoot. She scooped up Giovanni, brushed his long dark hair from his eyes, and kissed him on the cheeks. Pointing to the baby, she taught him a new word: *sorella*, sister. Generoso hugged his mama, the midwife. The baby girl's name, he told her, would be Rosina too. Bright-eyed baby Rose would soon be Rosina's shadow.

❦   ❦   ❦

That winter night in 2004, after driving Jenny home from her shift at the hospital, I squinted into the perfect lines of falling snow and traced them as far up as I could, until I was dizzy. Jenny had told me that I should call Melissa. *Call her. Just call her: she will know what to do.* I settled my eyes on a frosted tree across the yard to steady myself. Jenny said if I didn't want to tell her over the phone that I should go and see her in the morning. *Just drive over. You can't keep this a secret anymore.* The spots where the branches met the trunk were thick with snow. With a slight tug, the branches would break, a smooth snap and then a soundless landing. I wasn't going to say anything to anyone else.

A week passed, the snow kept coming. I was hoping to be stuck inside, buried to the rooftop. The furnace clicked on every few minutes, and the windows were iced over in the corners. The air slipped in through the old frames until Dad sealed them using a roll of plastic and a blow dryer. It was the coldest winter I could remember since elementary school, when it was too cold for the bus to start and too cold to go out for recess, a winter when we could stay inside and paint pictures and write stories, and I was happy.

This was the closest I had ever felt to Mom, even though I didn't tell her anything. I imagined her when she was seventeen. While the stigma of having a baby outside marriage had waned by 1975, the shame this pregnancy brought to her parents, and that her parents passed on to her, felt worse than the judgment of a stranger staring at her protruding belly. The social pressure to *give up* the baby was not as hurtful as her mother's pressure to give *her* the baby and pretend the pregnancy had never happened. Mom came from a long line of women who had many children, and she had inherited stories of motherhood and of surviving on nothing—no food, no sleep. Yet, she was the first child born to immigrant parents who wanted to build a faultless public life to show they belonged in Canada. As her pregnancy progressed, and as her body swelled, she felt pressed between the shame of having this baby alone and while so young and the fear that she would not be as capable, as mothering, as the women who had come before her. Either way, she felt she had a lot to prove. I knew now that Mom had needed to hear that her pregnancy was acceptable, but I suspect that she didn't hear anything like that.

Nanni Rose had only asked her if she was sure. Mom asked her to tell the news to her dad. In the months that followed, Mom found a job as a live-in nanny until, just before she was about to give birth, her aunt intervened on her behalf with a request for understanding. Nanni Rose then asked her to come back home and live in their basement. These snippets about Mom's pregnancy were filtered through Melissa, who, once pregnant herself, had asked her about it. Mom rarely gave up entire stories.

I tried to ask Mom anything about her experience. I'd look at her and practise the questions in my head. I could imagine her Catholic parents saying something about hell, sins, something about shame. Even if I told Mom that I could now understand what she had gone through, she would only nod, hug me, talk about a solution. Her parents' silence became her own.

The snow stopped. What had fallen had hardened into one crisp layer across the ground. I knew I had to go to the doctor; it had been almost three months since I had had a period. I had to drive down the highway into the city to the clinic. I had to pass by the familiar houses, fields, and farms, curve under the overpass and pass the golf course, and wonder if, on my way back, this world would look different. I had already imagined the trip several times, switching between possible outcomes, possible feelings. If I told Mom, she would make me go to the doctor. If I told Karl, we would go together. He'd sit there with me and wait. On the way, he'd adjust the mirrors, the fans. Reset the trip dial.

C I N Q U E

migrations arrows over oceans that chart the direction of movements

Young Rose spotted airplanes, flying low, over their farm. The massive grey planes, the first aircraft she'd ever seen, were like heavy, metal birds. Aside from the hum in her ears, the only proof Rose had seen of them was the trail of smoke lining the blue sky. She ran to the shed, where Rosina stood in the doorway, hand to forehead, looking up. Nanni Rosina explained that they were warplanes. At age six, all Rose knew about the war was that cousin Francesco had left Calabria to fight in it, but she didn't dare ask after him—last time she'd mentioned his name, she'd sent his mother, her aunt, into a crying fit. Rose imagined the airplanes zooming over the ocean, whooshing around the Earth and back, and wondered why so many neighbours had taken ships across the ocean when people could fly so much faster. She didn't dare ask about that either—leaving the village was a topic left to the adults. She'd heard stories about enormous navy ships. Four years earlier, in 1940, a naval battle had occurred off the Calabrian coast in the waters where she'd since dipped her toes. A British squadron and Italian squadron fired at one another, until, after much damage, Italy claimed victory.

Personal stories told and retold—of planes flying overhead, or of uniformed men demanding copper—scarcely touch on the political realities surrounding the isolated southern villages during the Second World War. Mussolini's Italy is the wall on which these snapshots hang. These personal images of family, captioned with hunger and poverty, are surrounded by bleak, more familiar images: a dictatorship allied with Nazi Germany, a country at war against Britain and France, a nation in combat against the USSR, and despite the millions of Italo-American migrants, an Italy in conflict with the United States and Canada. While the war raged around the isolated villages of Maione and Altilia, no family stories testify to the brutality experienced elsewhere in Italy and around the globe.

Beautiful Italian islands that excite western tourists and fill travel guides with windswept, soft-sand descriptions became places of imprisonment, banishment, and extreme violence. From 1926 to 1943, these islands with high rugged cliffsides, encircled by the sea, confined those deported by Mussolini's Fascist state. Once these places were full, the regime sent prisoners deemed less dangerous to isolated southern villages. While Altilia and Maione were certainly a part of the *Mezzogiorno*—the southern half of the Italian peninsula where prisoners were sent—no family stories tell of Mussolini's southern prisons.

❧ ❧ ❧

The house on the hill was full. By 1950, before anyone had left the country, Generoso and Michelina's family had grown to include five children: Giovanni, Rose, Vittorio, Maria, and Maurizio. Rosina, now in her late sixties, watched over the entire family and still managed to serve her community as a midwife.

At twelve, Rose helped with many of the chores and responsibilities to lessen the load on her Nanni Rosina. She scrubbed and squeezed the laundry in the river and carried the wet clothes up the hill to meet her grandmother, who took sheets and blankets from her arms. Rosina folded them over top of the line—half on one side, half on the other. Now that the war was over, people were moving again. Rosina realized that when everyone left for Canada there would be more space. Fewer people would mean less laundry. Just a few aprons. A dress pinned up by the shoulders. She imagined wooden pins clipped to an empty line. Generoso had spoken to some farmers who once travelled to Canada and he asked them for information about jobs, or if they had any connections. I imagine Rosina standing on the hill before a wire stretched across the sky, and can almost hear the tick, tick of clothespins being dropped into her basket.

One afternoon, in 1954, Rosina watched as her granddaughter Rose and grandson Vittorio collected acorns and pulled weeds. Vittorio sometimes joined Rose when he had finished work in the field or garden or when he wanted a break. He would sit with his back against a tree or roll seeds between his fingers while Rose filled the pails. As Rose was the second born, and oldest female, she understood responsibility. Rosina listened as Rose teased Vittorio about being lazy. He fired back that Rose should talk less and hurry up and fill those pails because there was plenty of other work to do. Then he got up, brushed his hands on the front of his pants, and left to snip the olive trees.

Rosina returned to the shed, where she had been feeding the chickens before taking a moment to listen to the mumbles of her grandchildren. As she scooped up a chicken, it squawked and flailed around while pecking the wire cage. A few feathers came off in her hand, and she shook them to the ground. They swayed in the air before finding new surfaces to land on. She spotted two eggs with smooth brown shells. She rolled both into her hand and cradled them. Food was scarce. The boys were eating more, especially at the end of long days working the farm—shaking olives from branches, pruning grapevines, and picking zucchinis. They would save her fistfuls of the yellow zucchini flowers to batter and fry. Rosina stood in the cool corner of the shed, where the wooden wallboards pressed together so firmly that no light slipped through, and reviewed her inventory of potatoes and carrots. Little remained after they had delivered the vegetables in Grimaldi, but their landowners had given Rose that cheese and Giovanni those mended shoes, so that was something.

Through the doorway, she spotted a man. He moved in and out of the trees like a ribbon in the wind. She squinted to see if he was one of her grandsons. After a few minutes, he attempted to cross the river. The stranger was a short young man with thick dark hair and a slender face.

"Buongiorno!" he called as he stepped onto the tree trunk that had been pulled across the water.

Rosina waved back and waited for him to cross. It was the young man from Altilia, come all this way in the thick of the afternoon. She suspected that he had come to speak to Rose. The water darkened the hem of his suit, and his hair, combed to one side, caught on some of the branches above. He swerved and swung.

He reminded her of their dog snapping at a wasp, and she looked away to stop herself from laughing.

He had made the suit himself, he told her, as he tugged at the sleeves. Rosina asked after his parents, and his aunt, whose baby she had recently delivered. All were well in Altilia, he explained. She was glad for the confirmation that his aunt and the baby were healthy. It had been a quick delivery. The chubby baby arrived a few days later than Rosina had expected, and he had let out a wail almost immediately. As the baby boy latched on to his mother's breast for milk, the two women gripped hands and whispered about the baby's clear skin.

Rosina looked at the young man before her, and remembered how she had tugged him into the world so many years before: he had the same head full of dark hair. She was often called to carry the babies she had delivered through the village to the church for their christenings—the baby's first public appearance. She led the processions, and this ritual knotted them together—the midwife and the child: she and Filippo.

Filippo asked if Rose was there, and if he could please speak with her. Rosina pointed to the trees at the edge of the field behind their house. He walked across the Russo's farmyard, kicking his feet out as he moved to keep his wet pants from sticking to his legs. When young Rose noticed Filippo in his suit she looked down at her black dress, which had belonged to her grandmother and was so long that it covered her feet. Rosina always told her to be modest, to wear long skirts, especially when working.

Rosina pretended to move buckets and baskets around, in and out of the shed, so that she could watch them. Filippo leaned against an oak that spread shade over the two like an umbrella. Rosina noticed he had crossed his feet at the ankles. Rose stood, hand on opposite elbow, and nodded. Filippo tugged at his sleeve and then outstretched his arm and pointed north. Rosina turned toward the shed, and when she reached the door, she glanced back at them. He leaned toward Rose and opened his arms, and Rose stepped forward between them. Rosina turned, wiped the sweat from her lip, and stepped into the cool darkness of the shed.

When Filippo left a few minutes later, he crossed back in front of the house to find the same spot at the river, to retrace his steps. Rosina told him to wait because she had something to give him. Filippo stood still with his hands in his lined pockets. She reached for the two eggs. The Ferrari family was one of the few that owned their own land in the area; they had enough food. She placed the eggs in his hands and wished him well.

Filippo kissed her on the cheeks, pressing his smooth face against her lined tough skin, and then slipped the eggs into his pocket. He was so happy, sure to have Rosina's blessing even if he didn't yet have Rose's. He jumped from rock to log across the river until he missed a step and splashed into the water. He heard the crunch of the shells against the rocks; when he stood up, the yolks dripped through his pocket.

"What did he come to say?" Rosina asked her granddaughter as she placed the buckets of acorns on a shelf in the shed.

"He told me that he is going to be leaving for Canada. He said that it is cold there. It looks like flour is spread over everything."

Rosina nodded, and then made her way to the house after tugging the shed door closed—latch to notch. She wasn't ready for the soil to split, to separate, the way she knew it was about to do.

❦   ❦   ❦

After the war, Italy estimated that it had close to two million unemployed citizens—Surplus Persons. The state maintained that a rapidly growing population was its main economic and social problem. Too many people. Too little food. In contrast, Canada had cities to build, a modern nation to construct, abundant food and resources, but not enough people. Canada needed railroads to boost its economy, to move goods and people from one coast to the other; it needed new workers to build thousands of new homes, new streets and highways, new schools and hospitals. That is what many Italian emigrants left their country to do.

The Intergovernmental Committee for European Migration (ICEM) began operations in February 1952, opening and widening areas of settlement around the world. Italy was one of the five main countries with which the ICEM worked, giving Italians new places to root their families, simultaneously fostering resettlement and ripping families apart.

Usually the men left first. They started new lives in places their families could only imagine through village stories. *The fields are flat and unending. In winter, your fingers get so cold that they feel like they are on fire.* Sometimes it was months or even years before the emigrants could afford to send one-way tickets to their wives or children. In the meantime, their families carried on at home because they had no choice. They drank from the same glasses, hung their clothes on the same lines, slept in the same beds. And waited.

Backstage, the international committee was organizing more exits: setting the scene for thousands of farewells throughout the 1950s in Italy and other western European countries. The committee helped emigrants across borders that had been cemented shut during the Second World War. Soon almost every Canadian city could boast a Little Italy.

Migration routes became global grooves. In just five years, the committee assisted 180,000 Italians to leave the country. The emigrants followed paths to Canada that previous generations had established decades earlier, to favoured destination cities such as Ottawa, Hamilton, Windsor, Sault Ste. Marie, Winnipeg, Edmonton, Calgary, and Vancouver. *Partono. Arrivano.* Nations had rarely co-operated in this way—the whole world shifting together—moving people across borders, expanding the meaning of home.

Except for Rosina who stood on the empty stage: arms cradled across her chest, eyes narrowed under the too bright sunlight, black dress billowing from the winds coiling off the sea. Her world became smaller and smaller with every goodbye. She could only imagine Canada, a huge expanse as far-reaching as her loss. She would be the only one in the family to remain in the Old Country. After Generoso left, the rest of her families' tickets would arrive one by one, in brown envelopes stamped with sepia-toned Eskimo kayaks and blue and white whooping cranes.

SEI

trap streets fictitious streets drawn on maps

In 2005, after a breakfast of sugared pastries and strong coffees in the port city of Genoa, we were in transit, moving straight across the top of Italy, then edging a little farther north, to Verona. Karl wedged sideways in his seat to get a full view of springtime Italy. I leaned into his back, my ribs hard against the armrest between us, our sweaty hands, palm to palm. It was hard to believe we'd made it through that long, cold winter. The train pulled past the rust-coloured fields of Liguria and Veneto, past clusters of dark cypress and their stretched-out, cone-shaped shadows, and past wooden buildings with roofs that sagged and walls that pressed outward, ready to lie flat under the blurry heat.

55

those long months before we left for Italy, I had watched the minute hand dawdle around the gas bar's clock until the end of each shift when I was another day closer to leaving. The Morinville gas bar was a tiny square in the corner of the parking lot of the town's newest grocery store, Extra Foods. I started work every day at 7:30 AM, just when the dog-food factory across the street began wafting fumes from a batch of kibble—a smell like raw meat left to thaw on the counter too long. One morning an older woman came in; while she was selecting a package of gum, she yelled in my direction, "Whoa! Smells like fried chicken out there. It's ghastly! Extra Foods must be havin' a special today."

Until the mid-morning rush, I would fold my arms across the counter and rest my head on them until the beep of the gas pump jolted me awake. I looked up and out the windows of the front of the store to see each familiar vehicle, and then matched the vehicle to the person, the person to the amount of fuel or brand of cigarettes each usually purchased. Light blue Dynasty: tall man who buys two packages of Peter Jackson Menthols. Mint-coloured Chevy truck: former childhood neighbour who buys forty dollars of premium fuel and two bottles of Aquafina.

A wall of thick glass separated me from the customers. Behind the glass, I flipped through guidebooks of Italy. I would put my finger on Portugal and my thumb on Newfoundland and pinch the space—the North Atlantic Ocean—squishing the land masses closer together. I highlighted restaurants in the *Lonely Planet* travel guide and made notes about the cities I wanted to visit. I especially wanted to stay in Verona. The guidebook's descriptions of this ancient city, with its landmarks that had first existed only in a fictional Verona, and were later imagined into reality, excited my imagination. *Lonely Planet*'s bible-thin pages told me that if I wandered the streets of Verona, I might believe the tragic story of Romeo and Juliet to be true. Just off Via G Mazzini, Verona's main shopping street, was the Casa di Giulietta, and the guidebook explained that if this theme appealed to me I could also visit the Tomba di Giulietta.

As I sat on my black swivel chair with my feet up on a garbage can, I imagined myself sitting at a little café, cobblestones beneath my feet. I saw myself sipping an espresso while I decided if passersby had descended from the Montagues or from the Capulets.

I vowed that on another trip, I would venture to the southern provinces where fewer spoke English, and fewer travelled, to the places where the true stories came from. I would meet the remaining descendants of the Russos, the Ferraris, and the Benincasas: my relatives. For now, like many new travellers, Karl and I would stay in the north and complete the Rome-Florence-Venice circuit. We would match the real streets to the squiggly black lines on our maps—and wander.

I planned to go to Calabria on a future visit. I imagined that down at the bottom of the peninsula, less than half a day away by train from the cities I'd be visiting this time, the trees would be the same as Nanni Rose had described, their house on the hill would still be standing, and the stones would still be placed evenly as footholds across the river.

I glanced up at the customers over the big red sticker plastered to the glass that read NO CASH ON PREMISES, slid their receipts under the glass window, and mouthed, "Thank you." I could never clearly hear anyone over the hum of the old computer. I counted the hours and recorded how much money I had saved selling cigarettes and ringing up peoples' diesel and gas.

One shift, I worked late to cover for another employee. At 9:30 PM I locked up for the night and pushed through the wind blowing against the side door. My truck had been sitting all day, but I noticed that my windshield and side mirrors had been cleared. Tire tracks in the fresh snow crossed one side of the parking lot, and footprints with small star cutouts pressed into the snow around my truck. I saw a white container on the hood and inside was a note that read, "I hope these cookies are as sweet as you are. Love, K." And I cried.

I drove over to Karl's house; we had heard there was going to be a meteor shower and had made plans to watch it. Karl was waiting in his car in the driveway. The warm air blasted through the fans and the scent of cardboard pine mixed with his sweet cologne. "Thanks for the cookies," I said and leaned over to hug him. He gripped the cold, plastic stick shift and lifted his palm. I slipped my hand under his and felt the clunk of the car click into reverse.

The tires crunched against the ruts of packed snow and ice as the car turned out of his parents' driveway. A mile or two down the road we bumped over the train tracks, like we always did, rattling the pennies in the cup holder. At the field—next to the graveyard— he turned off the engine.

The headlights, long through the dark, stretched across the empty field. He flicked them off. The car sank into the snow, settling with a groan against the ground. We climbed into the back seat, soaking the upholstery with our wet shoes.

I imagined what it would be like to have a baby seat strapped between us, and a future that we would map together out of necessity. As difficult as it would be to be young parents, some things would be more certain. We leaned our heads back and stared up through the wide back window. I thought that if we were patient, we'd see something.

Despite the daylight, the train's sway urged me to sleep. Passengers' voices, a rise and fall of words that I couldn't understand, became one solid hum. I slept until Karl said, "We have to get off."

"What? How long was I sleeping?"

"A while. I don't know what's going on. The train stopped. They are telling everyone to get off." Karl slid his backpack over his shoulders and held my straps for me to slide into mine.

"But we're not anywhere."

"We *are* somewhere. Just not Verona. There's a guy in a uniform saying something. See?" He pointed toward the train's accordion door where people were gesturing with sweeping hand motions, their white train tickets waving like small flags. The man was using his cigarette to point toward a brick building down the tracks.

"Uh. Perché?" I said to the man as I stepped off the train onto the platform. It came off my tongue as "perky" because I was in too much of a panic about getting off the train in the middle-of-nowhere to roll my Rs as recommended in the "basic phrases" section of the guidebook.

"Controllo di polizia," he said without looking at us.

"Police control?" repeated Karl as he headed toward the brick building, "I sure hope the police want to buy us new tickets."

We sat on the platform with backpacks as backrests and stretched our sandalled feet out across the smooth metal tracks. We worked on translating the euros to dollars to find out exactly how much our ride from Genoa to Milan, Milan to Nowhere, and Nowhere to Verona was costing us. We asked the woman issuing us new tickets why we had been forced to vacate the train. She smiled and recited some muffled words, which we couldn't even make out well enough to look up in our English–Italian travel dictionary.

"Well, either way, we aren't staying here," Karl whispered and slid our money under the glass. We grabbed the new tickets and then the woman leaned down to speak into the small hole in the glass. "Good. Bye."

Most people waited inside where it was air-conditioned, but we didn't want to miss the train. Some kids chased each other up and down the platform and some threw pebbles at the pigeons. The birds waddled and twitched but refused to leave their spots near the heaping garbage bins.

I practised saying "Perché?" and "Controllo di polizia" until Karl assured me that I sounded Italian and should now focus on expanding my vocabulary. While my blue-eyed, blond-haired, Swedish Canadian boyfriend didn't seem to mind that he could barely carry on a basic conversation in Italian, I felt ashamed that I couldn't summon the language I felt I should know—the language I had so often heard my grandparents speak to each other and to relatives while I was growing up.

❧   ❧   ❧

"I am going to watch the tella-vezi-onah," said Nonno as he grabbed his glass of orange juice off the table and tucked *The Edmonton Journal* under the arm of his plaid shirt.

Nanni laughed, and her thick grey and white curls bounced on her round shoulders.

"He makes everything sound Italian. That man. He does not know the Italian word for it. Don't try to learn Italian from him!" Nanni laughed.

Nonno turned to me, scrunched up his dark eyebrows, creating olive creases on his forehead, and, with one finger in the air, asked, "What do you put in egg salad sandwiches?"

"Mayonnaise, Nonno."

He smirked under his perfectly trimmed dark moustache and shook his finger. "No. No. Mayo-naziah! See? It's easy."

When I was in elementary school in Morinville, I savoured sleepovers at Nanni and Nonno's place in Edmonton, a sharp right off Yellowhead Trail at 50th Street. I would wake up early to the smell of sugar, eggs, coffee, and fresh air. I skipped my bowl of Lucky Charms and Saturday morning cartoons and sat at their kitchen table waiting for French toast made with bread from the Italian bakery. Nanni dusted icing sugar over the top. She wiped her powdery fingertips across her apron and then smiled at me with her hands on her round hips.

When she moved though the kitchen, I'd look up at the wooden cupboards and wonder what was hidden in there, tucked behind the jars of spices with orange lids; everyone said that she must have secrets. She didn't write any recipes down. She'd always say, "They're all in my memory, Jessica. A little of this, a little of that, and there you go!"

When the sun shone through the peach curtains over the sink, they looked like they were made of tissue paper. The window was usually open to offer air to the sprouting tomato and basil plants on the windowsill.

This was the kitchen that Nanni cooked in the most, but downstairs she had a second kitchen, another set of drawers filled with silverware, plates, and glasses and another table that she used when the whole family was over. She always stuffed both ovens full of lasagnas, hams, and turkeys; she would boil soups and potatoes on both stoves; she would pack one of the fridges with plates of *pitaletta*, her special cooked broccoli wrapped in dough.

Underneath the stairs, Nonno had built a roomful of wooden shelves. This room with a low ceiling held a wide freezer, and was lit by a yellow light bulb yanked on by a chain. Every shelf was piled with food: packages of penne noodles, shell pasta, linguini, spaghetti, tortellini, and cans of pickled vegetables, stuffed olives, peppers, and jams. There were packages of spices with labels I couldn't read; the bags had little red, white and green flags on them. When Nanni was cooking, I offered to go down into the food room to get whatever she needed. I pretended I was in an Italian grocery shop, the jingle of the metal chain became the bell signalling my entrance, and I mumbled words with *-oni* and *-ee* endings to the "cashier" as I was leaving.

While Nanni cooked the slices of French toast, I ran my finger along the edges of her fancy plates; I listened, trying to gather some words to use in my grocery shop.

Nanni curled the white phone cord around her wrist and let it drop to the ceramic tile. The tick, tick of the cord as she moved around the kitchen, along with the steady drip of coffee, mixed with words that came from her belly, words that filled the room with booming *ahhs* and *onis*. Sometimes she would stand still, hold the phone between her shoulder and ear, and look out at the garden. She would move her hands up and down with her words, or pinch off the dry basil leaves and put them in the sink. Sometimes she tied a new floppy bow with the apron strings, but she never stopped talking. I heard names, long and loud, like Maa-ri-ah and Toe-nee-noo.

I took small bites of my breakfast and sipped my pulpy orange juice because I wanted to stay, seated there, in the middle of it all. When I was finished pushing my last forkful of bread through the pool of syrup on my plate, Nanni would cover the phone receiver and lean toward me as she plopped another piece of toast down. "Eat! Eat! You are too skinny, my bella," she'd say before returning to her conversation.

I watched her words travel through the wires to Italy, spiral around like the plastic cord and twist into some faraway kitchen. I imagined the windows in that kitchen would be open because someone wanted to feel the sea breeze, but then Nanni could have been talking to her sister-in-law or brother in Edmonton. For me, those words, whirling around, always made their way across the ocean, always made their way to Italy.

❧　❧　❧

Karl adjusted his backpack backrest and rolled up the sleeves of his white cotton T-shirt to avoid tan lines. "At least we are in the middle-of-Italy-nowhere in the north."

"Why? Because the guidebook said there was better food?"

"Less seafood, less mafia, and more Engli . . . there it is!"

We found spots at the front of the train. There were no seats in front of us, just a picture of an escape route, and we were able to stretch out. When we neared Verona, I was half asleep. The toss and tug of the train cradled me again. I was thinking about what Nanni told me before I left: to be careful. She went through her usual list of precautions on account of the bad people in the world and explained that I should not trust just anyone. As I was leaving my grandparents' house, Nanni had hugged me, her soft short body a warm cushion. I rested my head over top of hers. Then she held me away from her, her hands on my arms, and looked right at me, "My Jessica. I would never go back. Never. Nope!"

Karl and I arrived in Verona in time for a late dinner. The tour of Casa di Giulietta would have to wait until morning. I stepped onto the platform and moved from the train station to the bus depot with the address of our hotel in hand after an entire day in transit. As I lay in bed that night in fair Verona, wrapped in a white sheet in the stifling room, I wondered why Nanni had said that. I thought that it must be because her Italy had Rosina in it. When she imagined this country, it probably still did.

She could probably still see her Nanni Rosina carrying a basket of fruit under her arm or washing the vegetables. Maybe she imagined something more intimate, a kiss on the forehead before bed or a warm hand pressed against her shoulder the day that her dad left for Canada. Maybe it was her Nanni Rosina's words that she remembered from the day that she and her brother left too. Those words exchanged in their Calabrese dialect would be forever foreign to me, a language I could never learn in university.

A part of me worried that I might enter into my own family myth, the place where our stories came from, the place we lay *our* scene and that I wouldn't recognize anything. What if all of the family landmarks, those spots where the stories circle around, were fictional? Either way I promised that I'd make it to Maione.

SETTE

routes the pathways and rest spots along the way

It is 1952, time for Generoso to leave. In the days leading up to his departure, which would be the first goodbye of many, Rosina relied on steady demands—yanking up potatoes, uprooting this- tles, pulling herself up before daylight to bake bread—to keep her days together. She listened as Michelina reminded the children that they'd see their father in time, that sooner or later they would all end up in Edmonton. And I can imagine that overhearing the word *Edmonton*—a hard word, a series of heavy sounds—would create a full stop. A pause at the stove or at the woodpile. A moment for Rosina to rest her hand on Rose's shoulder.

As Generoso would have to first make his way to Naples, I

imagine that he left in the morning and that Rosina didn't have the agony of a day punctuated by that goodbye. I imagine that Rosina gave Michelina and Generoso the space to talk, to solidify plans and say their temporary farewell. She waited for the moment to say her permanent one. Generoso, her thirty-eight-year-old son, was her youngest—her baby boy, and though she'd held so many babies, crouched to catch them in her hands, she remembered cradling him, the curl of his body in her arms, especially on those long, lonely nights after Giovanni died. He grew up to look so much like his father. She didn't have a picture of her husband, but she could see him when she looked into her son's face: everyone could. And, as her family would resettle, she would be left to remember this day of goodbyes and their faces—Giovanni's and Generoso's. And their eyes so dark that she couldn't see their pupils—so dark that she could see her face reflected in Generoso's as she stepped back, her hands still on his shoulders, and smiled as she wished him safe travels.

It is 1952, time for Generoso to leave. In the days leading up to his departure, Rose noticed that everyone seemed busy: her dad, packing up his things and talking about money; her mom, discussing plans and verifying dates; her Nanni, cooking meals for the family and the neighbours who stopped by, and washing and folding her dad's clothes. Everyone was talking about *Edmonton,* a word that scared her, a word that told her that after her dad earned money and sent their tickets, she'd have to say goodbye to Nanni Rosina too. The word *Edmonton* reminded her that Nanni Rosina was staying behind. When Nanni Rosina pressed her warm hand down on her shoulder, she leaned back into her and took a moment.

Rose watched as her dad pulled Nanni Rosina close. Sometimes, it was easy to forget that even her dad was a child once, and that even though he was an adult now, he probably still liked having a mother to take care of him. She was glad that her mom was staying in Calabria with her, and that when her dad sent her a ticket to go to Canada, her mom would come soon after—she was happy that they wouldn't have to be apart long. Her dad had a tight look on his face when Nanni Rosina stepped back. Rose didn't know when he would see his mother again, but didn't want to ask. Nanni Rosina didn't cry, but as soon as Rose stepped forward to say goodbye to her father, she did. He reminded her that she'd get to ride a ship over with her younger brother Vittorio, and that he'd be waiting for her. By the time she could find her voice again and yelled, "Arrivederci, Papà!" he was already too far away to hear her.

"Non sará tanto tempo," Nanni Rose said. It won't be long.

Rosina had heard the plan: Generoso would make his way from Halifax to Edmonton, where the family would eventually reunite.

He would send for his oldest son, Giovanni, just as soon as he had saved enough money, so that he could also get a job in Edmonton. After that, when he had saved up some more, he would send for Rose and Vittorio. Once he had enough money, he'd send for Michelina and their two youngest children, Maria and Maurizio. And maybe once they were settled in Edmonton and had bought a house, they would even try for another baby—a baby that Rosina wouldn't be there to deliver, a baby born in a hospital.

A few of Michelina's older cousins had already left. They'd heard there were jobs on Canadian railroads and some other construction jobs for the city. There was talk among some wives still in Calabria that many of the men planned to stay in Edmonton, that they'd form a new community there. Michelina told Rosina that the Italians went to worship together, and she felt better knowing that her family would have people to talk to and pray with.

That didn't make it any easier to watch Generoso leave to a place she would only ever know through village stories. Michelina relayed what she'd heard from other migrants' wives: a cousin told her that Edmonton was a long, flat city, in the winter people only left their houses when they had to. She had heard that the snow was thick and that sometimes it was so heavy it would snap a shovel. Rosina imagined looking out the window of a new house and seeing footprints across their snow-covered yard like fingerprints pressed into dough. She imagined tracing Generoso's thick bootprints when he left for work, and following him through a white glow.

Soon, as the neighbouring farmers began to lock up, to follow cousins to new countries, the flow of the river would change. For years, farms had fed into the river system as workers watered terraced grapevines, nourished the purple fruit, plump between their fingertips. Soon, the water would slow down. The hillsides would develop deep cracks. There would be dry, bud-less vines against wooden posts and strings of wire.

❦   ❦   ❦

In early 2010, five years after travelling to Italy with Karl, I started planning another trip: while sitting cross-legged on my living room carpet, staring at my gaping, wide-mouthed laptop on the coffee table, the sound of my fingers on the keys tapped against the silence of the night. The more I read about southern Italy as the hours scrolled by, the more I realized that I'd need a translator—my godfather, Uncle Roberto, perhaps. I made a note to call him: trip to Calabria, summer 2010? The websites were full of links that took me all over the Internet: language sites with basic phrases I tried to memorize, snapshots of rocky beaches, and pages of statistics about the declining population in the south. I navigated my way to pictures of Karl, clicking through folders until I found gelato-faced, knock-off-handbag versions of myself leaning into my near-sunburned now-ex-boyfriend. I looked up emails we'd exchanged about our northern tour: we'd watched a documentary about Pompeii and the eruption of Mount Vesuvius in 79 AD and had opened a shared savings account. In other messages, we had plotted the years ahead, and imagined what it would be like to pass milestones together. I felt a quiet guilt, some ache in my gut that I couldn't remedy, each time those moments played out in my life without him: a revision he hadn't been consulted about. I resisted sending him a message because even though I was going back to Italy, something we had promised to do together, everything had changed. What would I say? When I eventually pulled myself up and into bed, I trusted that in the morning I'd be glad I didn't send him an unexpected email that he likely wouldn't answer.

One night, as I tossed with the whirl of foreign words in my mind, I thought of Generoso's journey. He had sailed from Naples to Halifax, then travelled to Edmonton. For two long weeks, the rhythm of the ship's rise and fall against the force of the Atlantic had buoyed *Mam-ma* in his heart. It's easy to see him, fingers laced together, elbows on the railing of the ship, staring forward and waiting. I know that Generoso's journey is part of a much larger story, and I wonder about the shared experience connecting individual migrants. In the morning, I put the laptop on the kitchen counter, made sure my inbox was empty, and began another search as the coffee dripped into the pot and warmed the room. As I clicked through websites about the emigrations from southern Italy, I soon saw my lone great-grandfather standing beside a long line of men smoking, spitting over the rail, and discussing plans.

I clicked through websites until I discovered the work of Franc Sturino, an academic who has written extensively about the history of Calabrians in Canada. As I moved down the page I realized that his research was comprehensive. I balanced my laptop on the palm of one hand, carried my mug of steaming coffee and cream in another, and shuffled to my bedroom. Nestling back into bed I perched my laptop on my bare knees. Sturino says that Italian migration from 1870 to 1970 represents one of the major diasporas of the modern age. In a single century, twenty-six million Italians left *il loro paese*, their homeland. That means twenty-six million migrant stories: people shoulder to shoulder on ships sailing over the sea. This mass of people is comparable to the entire population of Canada in the mid-twentieth century. In the 1950s, when this Italian emigration gained momentum, Canada's population was only thirteen million—the country certainly had the space for newcomers.

I leaned back into my pillows and up at the spackled ceiling. I imagined that the two weeks it took for Generoso to arrive in Canada felt like months, especially at night while in the cheapest of the cabins in the bottom of the ship, he heard the waves slapping and surging. Many Calabrians made this same trip; thousands switched off their bedside lights in their cabins and listened to the water. Further on, Sturino explains that there were two major waves of emigration: between 1900 and the First World War and then from 1950 to 1970. Early emigration involved fathers, husbands, and brothers in search of money to make a better life. For our family, this early history is filled out by the story of Rosina's older brother—no one could recall his name—who left Calabria before the First World War and died somewhere in America. He died there in an accident—a train or a car.

The second wave of emigration, the wave that Generoso, Michelina, and their children were a part of, was more permanent. Entire families left and didn't come back. It is tempting to believe that because migration, and, with that, separation, happened so often during this twenty-year period, it was somehow easier on those saying the goodbyes. When I slow down and imagine one of these goodbyes, like those scenes in 1952, I realize that regardless of the frequency that people left or their reasons why—political, cultural, or otherwise—for many, these moments signalled tremendous losses. Italian migrants' return rate from Canada was the lowest in the world. Generoso didn't return for twenty years, and when he did, his mother was dead.

In small Calabrian villages like Maione and Altilia, this mass migration left houses abandoned and fields untilled. In some instances, for particularly well-situated pieces of land, some families took over emigrants' old houses and well-worn jobs. Villages shifted and shrunk. Eighty percent of Italian migrants left from provinces south of Rome—places like Puglia, Basilicata, and Calabria—which alleviated some of the hardships created by too many people depending on too little work. Despite mass emigration, Calabria is still one of Italy's most rural and least industrialized regions, the income per capita is less than half the national average, and people are still leaving.

I spent the rest of the morning clicking through websites with black-and-white images of those who had left. I read captions about where the emigrants found employment in America, Canada, and Australia, about who they married and their contributions. My mind turned to Rosina. Her children and grandchildren, not unlike those in these digital images, belonged in these settlement stories. I can imagine Generoso as the male sojourner in Sturino's historical accounts of emigration, but what of Rosina, a matriarch to a line of migrants?

❧   ❧   ❧

After learning about leaving, I became more interested in arrival stories. I spent a few more nights in the living room, in slippered feet and baggy sweatpants, with my laptop casting a white light over my hands. I'd become so used to reaching for a warm drink that I had to have a cup of steaming water beside me to fuel my search: after a few nights, I realized that caffeine was, in part, to blame for my tossing at night, for the dreams of boarding ships that bobbed over dark water and never arrived anywhere.

I'd heard the stories of Generoso's arrival and about how quickly the city had spread out. The family stories, put up against the facts I'd been finding about the journey to Canada, and Edmonton in the 1950s, helped me to imagine what the first few days in Edmonton might have been like: Generoso stood on the snowy bank of the North Saskatchewan River that cut the city in two and could still feel a sway within his body, an uneasy feeling in his gut. Generoso and his fellow *paesani* rented places north of the river, on the eastern edge of the city. Steel trusses were in place for a new bridge that in one year's time would span the gushing North Saskatchewan. Some Italians lived in the town of Beverly near the main roadway, the paved Yellowhead Trail that stretched east to west. The Yellowhead took its name from the trail of a nineteenth-century Métis fur trader, Pierre Bostonnais, nicknamed Tête Jaune for his blond hair; the modern road crossed prairie and parklands and entered a mountain pass through the Rockies. Inside Edmonton, it was a gritty concrete speedway: a flat, unending strip of grey unlike the winding trails and cobble fishhook streets that carved Calabria.

Generoso began work for the Canadian National Railroad before he had time to settle his seasickness or learn to navigate this new life. Along with other immigrants, he'd help to continue to bridge Canadian cities, towns, and pit stops. He ignored the blisters building up on his already calloused hands; he worked long hours, alongside other southern Italians, despite the sting of the prairie winter on his face. The cold went through his clothes and into his bones.

Most of the Italian immigrants that Generoso met came from the southern regions, and together they suffered through the bitter first few years to save and send for their families. An online search of "Italians in Edmonton" turned up an article from *The Edmonton Journal* about one man, Peter Batoni, who came to be a well-known immigrant in the city. I had heard about him from my grandparents. Peter had a different story: he studied architecture in Switzerland, and then moved to London, where he met a Canadian who suggested he go to Montreal. From there, he eventually made his way to Edmonton. He established one of the largest construction companies in North America and employed immigrants, including Generoso's son-in-law and nephews.

Batoni was considered a pioneer in pre-cast concrete structure, and one of his most recognizable projects, an Edmonton hockey arena originally named the Coliseum, was constructed close to the district where most Italians settled. The ancient

Romans, credited with the invention of concrete, created structurally complex buildings, including two of Rome's main attractions: the Pantheon, with its concrete dome ceiling and perfect oculus centre, and the Colosseum, with its arches that still draw thousands of visitors. When Edmonton's Coliseum—a massive concrete building with a series of flat rectangular panels along the outside of its circular frame—was completed in 1974, it was regarded as the best arena in North America, a hockey palace for a city in love with the game, and also a concert venue. Many immigrants had worked to create this landmark. A North American drugstore chain bought the naming rights and the Coliseum was renamed Rexall Place, eliminating all immediate signifiers of its Italian connections.

I kicked off my slippers, creaked open the closet, and pulled up my knee-high boots. I had driven past Rexall Place dozens of times but never really stopped to look at it. My tires turned against the slush, kicking up tiny rocks and chunks of frozen muck. To my right, as I drove over Capilano Bridge, I could see the bright blue lights that illuminated Rexall Place from the ground up. Pylons dotted the cleared sidewalks, indicating where to turn into parkades. On other drives, I had seen people in reflective vests wave batons to coax people into their lots. To my left a rundown restaurant advertised steak on a hand-painted sign, and a bright mural on the Axe Music store completed the collage. I'd always thought it was an ugly stretch of the city. Edmonton's Coliseum was a far cry from the perfectly crumbling arches of the Roman amphitheatre where I had tucked myself under Karl's arm while wearing too big sunglasses and where we snapped a million photos because the late afternoon light had been perfect.

I pressed my breaks and bumped forward over an icy patch until I came to a complete stop. With Batoni's Coliseum in my rear-view mirror, I wondered about the divide between young immigrants seeking adventure and those like Generoso who had arrived to work. I had read about north–south politics, about the idea of two Italys, *due Italia*. Vito Teti, a Calabrian Canadian social historian like Sturino, offers depth to the discussion of southern Italian emigration. He explains the strained north–south relationship. *Due Italia* is a notion that suggests the superiority of the people of the north over the people of the south. The south is characterized as agrarian and pastoral, and poorer, while the north is full of industrial activity based, in part, on the exploitation of southern resources. When Generoso laid his head down on the first night in a tiny rented room in Edmonton, not far from where the Coliseum would be erected, I doubt he was considering adventure. Instead, survival.

❧ ❧ ❧

By spring 1955, an important moment on the family timeline, Generoso had saved enough money to bring Rose and Vittorio to Canada. In Calabria, Rosina squeezed the thick envelope and ran her fingers over the stamps. Unlike the other letters sent to the house on the hill, she wanted to open this one in private. She waited until the house was empty: Michelina and Rose had left for the market, and everyone else was busy in the field. She sat at the kitchen table with Generoso's letter. She pressed her nail down along the side seam and then ripped down the crease. She shook out three papers: one letter from Generoso, just a few words that she couldn't read in the middle of the page, and two third-class tickets for the SS *Andrea Doria* that looked like the ticket that Generoso had purchased for himself. The tickets, with numbers and letters stamped in thick black ink and filled with lined boxes, were for Rose and Vittorio.

> Westbound. April 25, 1955. Naples
> to Halifax and New York. Arrival in
> Halifax May 4, 1955.

She put the papers in a pile. She brushed some breakfast crumbs off the table, pushed her chair in, and went to rest in bed. She had known for a long time that the day would come when her life would be divided. Her entire life had been spent in Calabria, and now every member of her family was moving across the Atlantic. *Due Italia.*

Rosina's ticket would never arrive. When Generoso had asked, she told him that she could not go. He knew her answer before he voiced the question. She couldn't survive the two weeks at sea. Except when she was needed as a midwife, she had been staying close to home. Sometimes, she had to use walls, beds, trees, and posts to steady herself. Her head was fuzzy, the world in her periphery squeezed in and out. Rose had been developing the same sickness. They could feel the world turning. Rose would feel sick to her stomach if she ran too fast through the field or jumped too high off a stump or porch. Rosina worried that the trip to Canada would be hard for her granddaughter and she prayed for her safety.

Rosina never saw the ship's long black body or its smooth white railings and square windows because she was too dizzy to see her grandchildren off in Naples. And Rose never saw the ship's three outdoor swimming pools that she had heard about. She spent days with her head over the side of the bed vomiting into a bucket on the floor.

The SS *Andrea Doria* became a symbol of national pride upon its maiden voyage in 1953. Named after a sixteenth-century general from Genoa, the Italian port city in the north, the ship was marketed as the greatest, latest, and fastest Italian liner. In the war that had just ended, Italy had lost much of its merchant fleet. What had not been destroyed was used to pay Allied forces seeking war reparations. While the country's economy had collapsed, the *Andrea Doria* and another vessel, the *Cristoforo Colombo*, were commissioned as a sign to the world that Italy was recovering and was still a strong international force.

The *Andrea Doria* carried Rose, Vittorio, and hundreds of other Italian passengers from Naples to Halifax just fifteen years after Italy had declared war on Canada on June 10, 1940. That evening in 1940, Canada's prime minister, Mackenzie King, had addressed his small nation over CBC Radio: he announced that the minister of justice had authorized the Royal Canadian Mounted Police (RCMP) to intern residents of Italian origin whose activities gave grounds for belief, or who raised reasonable suspicion, that in a time of war they might endanger the safety of the state. These Italian Canadians were deemed enemies. To contain perceived internal threats, Canada locked up the suspects in an internment camp in Petawawa, Ontario, and forced others, who had been classified as threats outside the camps, to report regularly to the RCMP. The authorities forced prisoners to wear blue clothes with red full moons on the back, and locked them behind barbed-wire fences under bright security lights as if they were common criminals. Only a few of these people had been members of the Italian Fascist Party. Under Canada's War Measures Act, hundreds of innocent people were locked up even though they had never been charged with an offence against the state.

In the United States, 228 of the 6 million Italian Americans were briefly interned, but the situation in Canada was darker. Of the 112,000 Italians living across Canada at the beginning of the Second World War, 30,000 Italians were cast as "resident aliens" and 600 of them were interned. One personal story tells of a prisoner in the isolated camp in Petawawa who was interrogated about his allegiances. He proclaimed that, if called, he would be willing to join the Canadian army—willing to fight on behalf of Canada. A week after his release from imprisonment, he was called to fight. For him, this war was not narrated by the conflicts between nations but instead by a consuming fear that he would be forced to fight against his own brother, his blood, a member of the Italian army, who had not migrated to North America.

After the war, the borders reopened. Italians could immigrate again, but enemy labels still existed—now harsh whispers. While the boycotts and bans on Italian businesses and products were lifted, the reputations of some immigrants had been damaged. The Italian language could be spoken in public once again, although many people still feared using their primary language. A new wave of Italian immigrants supplied the now-booming economy with the hordes of foreign workers that the country required to develop its resources. For many, the nostalgia for Italy that had once been expressed through social clubs—a membership that had become cause to imprison—became part of a complex relationship with Canada. Where did they belong?

Just over a year after Rose and Vittorio were reunited with their father and brother in Edmonton, the *Andrea Doria*, carrying more than seventeen hundred passengers and crew, collided with the Stockholm, a small post-war liner heading home to Sweden. The two ships, running a parallel course, crashed in the dark ocean. Forty-six passengers on the *Andrea Doria* were killed.

Rosina, at home in Maione, looked up at the stars that night before she fell asleep, up at the tiny pinheads of light, and moved the rosary beads between her thumb and forefinger. Passengers hurried over the railing into the lifeboats and into the water. The next morning, as Rose and Vittorio woke up to the bright spring morning in Edmonton, the *Andrea Doria* capsized and sank to the bottom of the ocean.

❧   ❧   ❧

In 1972, three years after Rosina's death, Generoso would again cross the ocean that divided his worlds, this time by aircraft, and re-enter the place now known for its exits. I imagine him walking over cone-shaped shadows of cypress trees, the dark clusters we saw out the train window on our way to Verona. I see him walking up the hill to the house where he once lived with Michelina and Rosina. Wheat stalks, tall and brittle, snap beneath his feet the way they snap under mine when I walk across the fields of my father's childhood farm in Mearns, Alberta. But then, it may have been a field of yellow broom, or a patch of cyclamen blooms bordered by lemon trees.

With my uncle Roberto's confirmation that we would travel to Calabria in just a few months, I thought of my great-grandfather's return trip. I examined Google Maps, web-translated genealogy sites, checked the value of the euro, and wondered what it was like for Generoso to make his way back home. He'd no doubt lost touch with many of his remaining relatives, and while I could easily send an email to the archivist of a southern Italian history site, or to a village's *comune*, or town hall, to ask what documentation I should bring with me, he suffered a disconnection upon arriving in Edmonton that would have diminished in the Internet era. The multiple ways of staying in touch afforded by technology, embedded in my everyday, make it difficult to imagine such separation.

I had only heard one story about Generoso's return trip—it was as if he slipped into the place of his past and then back again to his garden in Edmonton. The story was about how Rosina's photo, recovered from a dump—proof of miracles—made its way to Edmonton. He arrived in Maione, and went to visit Sisina, the woman who had helped to care for Rosina at the end of her life.

He wanted to see his mother's belongings. While Rosina had been dead for three years, Sisina had decided, just a few days earlier, to clear out the older woman's belongings: she lived in a small house and didn't have room to store Rosina's stuff. Generoso immediately went to the dump and began ripping into the bags of garbage. In some versions, he rips into four bags—plastic and paper tumble out until he has it. I want to believe he knew that it was the one. He peels the black plastic and sees her face, holds the picture to his chest. In other versions of the story, he finds the photograph in the first bag he grabs. Either way, on this trip, he did bring home that picture.

I called Nanni Rose to ask what she knew about her late father's trip. Her voice was faint, so I turned up the volume on my phone. She explained that she had just woken up from a nap and that she wasn't feeling well. She murmured that she'd had a blood transfusion, but, like my mom often does, downplayed how sick she was feeling. Nanni Rose, now in her early seventies, speaking in a quiet voice—usually booming—frightened me. I pictured her seated in the kitchen with a mug of warm tea cradled between her palms. The phone rests on her shoulder, and she presses it into her cheek. As she talked about feeling sick, all of her words ran together.

"I swept the floor earlier today so I must be better. So, what can I tell you about Rosina?" she asked, her voice a little more lively as she drew out the "ahh" of Rosina's name.

"Nothing, Nan," I answered, aware that I had already collected most of the memories that she was willing to share. "I am actually wondering about your dad's trip home that you mentioned a while ago. If you know anything . . ."

"Ah, yes. Dad's trip. He went back, it was a few years before your sister, Melissa, was born and let's see . . . thirteen years before you were born."

Melissa, as Nanni's first grandchild, is often used as a marker: the time before she was a grandmother and the time after. Nanni Rose explained that Generoso went for a visit, just to see what the villages had become. She keeps a photo of her dad on a small table in her dining room and I wondered if she was looking over at it. In it, Generoso wears a grey sweatshirt and is crouched down next to his huge red tomatoes. The green leaves and thick stalks are tied back with pantyhose, and he smiles, stretching grey and white stubble up his cheeks. This is the Generoso that I place in a patch of cyclamen, a landscape I know through the work of Calabrian Canadian poets, or sometimes in a field in Mearns, a landscape I know through a childhood in Alberta: years spent yanking dandelions and braiding wheat-stalk bracelets.

Nanni Rose reminded me, as she always does, that he was a good father and that he had worked hard his whole life—in Calabria and in Alberta—to provide for his family. This *whole life* sentence was something I could recite, a line from our family history that we'd all heard. I nodded, though I was on the phone, because I knew what came next: she explained that he saved money and sent it back to his mother so that he could care for her even if he was not there.

"You know. It *was* a hard life. Dad eventually got Alzheimer's, and he would think he saw little kids in his house. The kids were always working. Most of the time he was okay, but sometimes he even thought he was back home in Italy."

I wondered if those kids were his brown-eyed sons with dirt on their pants and palms from a day of turning the soil in the field in Maione, or if he saw himself pushing the metal plow, just after he had learned to walk without gripping his mother's hand. It seemed especially cruel—an immigrant with Alzheimer's—for a man who had likely already struggled to remember a distant home and people.

"Dad did what he could to earn money for his family. He even built a bridge in Maione, a big one. But it's probably gone now. Maybe you could find it?"

"I'll look for it, Nan."

She instructed me that when I have children I should tell them about the bridge. I should tell them that he used a wheelbarrow and lifted boulders and that he fit the boulders together and then secured them with concrete. Everything was done by hand.

I needed to go to the Italy that my family came from. On my

first trip, I had travelled by train through the northern countryside between destination cities, snapping photos in front of the Casa di Giulietta and Michelangelo's David. Yet, once I returned to Alberta, I realized I needed to follow my great Nonno Generoso.

"Maybe it is still there . . . And, Jessica, it really didn't get that much easier when Dad came to Edmonton, you know? The railroad. The men put down those tracks. Most of them were immigrants. But at least when we got here that horrible voyage was behind us. Those waves. Those nauseating waves."

I waited a moment, sure Nanni was about to tell the story—her goodbye with Rosina that day in 1955—a scene that I'd come to imagine so fully since it had often bookended memories of the Old Country. Instead, she said she loved me, she'd talk to me soon, and then she hung up.

I imagine it was hot on that day in April when she left Italy—heat hangs the way heavy feelings do, heat slows things down. I had watched the blurry scene play out every time Nanni Rose told the story. While I set the stage myself—a cross-section of Calabria, Maione as an island, the farm an entire world—Nanni's voice, still with a trace of an accent, narrates. I imagine that the warmth of the afternoon curled the leaves to a crisp, that it drew thirsty branches to the ground, and that everything around them slouched under the weight of that day. Rose curled into Rosina, begged her to come along though she knew her grandmother would not leave Maione. When I imagine them standing there: granddaughter and grandmother, Nanni Rose's voice wraps around the scene: *The hardest thing I ever had to do was leave her. I knew I would never see her again. I would never be back there. She raised us. My mom was working, but Nanni Rosina was like a mother.* She studied Rosina's face, the shadows beneath her deep-set eyes— mother, midwife, matriarch.

O T T O

scatterplot points dispersed across a map
connected by a single line

Those days, when I was in elementary school in Morinville, it was
always Dad behind the wheel as we cruised along the Yellowhead
to visit Nanni and Nonno. The drive in from Morinville—just north
of Edmonton, where Mom grew up and traded her prosciutto
sandwiches for peanut butter and jam, and just east of Mearns,
where my Irish German dad spent his youth riding tractors and
swinging down from the hay loft on heavy ropes—seemed far
away from Nanni's and Nonno's home.

Mom, the perpetual passenger due to her motion sickness,
was the storyteller. Since her hands were free, she used them to

animate her stories. She'd tell us that if she looked at the road, the yellow line moved from side to side; then she would turn to us and slither her hands through the air. Mom would press a finger against the windshield, somewhere above the line of the road, and say, "If I look out here, at the horizon or higher, everything stays in place."

When I felt queasy during the forty minutes in the back seat—squished between my brothers—I'd look for the spot on the windshield to calm my spinning stomach. Dad would joke that we should see Mom ride a bicycle. While imitating her, he swerved between the lanes, sending my stomach on another round. Mom would slap him on the arm and swear in Italian, as if swearing wasn't so bad if it wasn't in English.

Once, when I was eight, Mom told us that she had attended Queen Elizabeth High School in the city. She said that the school had more students than all the schools in Morinville put together. I asked how big the playground was. I imagined rows and rows of monkey bars and tire swings. I could tell my younger brother, wide-eyed, was trying to imagine it too. When she said that high schools didn't have playgrounds, my endless play area turned into an empty field and the sand pits into dry grass. I felt content with Notre Dame Elementary: my tiny blue and white school, with its twisty yellow slide and a wooden bridge that wiggled from side to side. My school sat safely in a small town without any traffic lights.

When Mom told us stories, I wished I could see all of the

places she described. The Yellowhead Trail's thick cement walls blocked any view of Edmonton until we rushed past Beechmount Cemetery where the walls gave way to a metal fence. I would stare though the fence's honeycomb holes at the black stones that looked like oversized chess pieces. In the wintertime, dirty mounds of snow and sand would collect along the sides of the road, and we would slosh through them in our red minivan. I imagined that if I flew above the cemetery it would look like a chessboard. As a child, I associated Edmonton with carsickness, cement, and the Beechmount chess game perfectly sized for God.

When I was a little older, Mom told us that one night when she was twenty, she had been walking across a field on 54th Street to get to her apartment. I've seen pictures of her at this age, and it's easy to imagine her stepping out of the Polaroid frame: Lucianna with thick black curls, round brown eyes, and always wearing heels—however uncomfortable and impossible the angles, as long as they were in fashion. She moves in a diagonal line across the flat ground, with a big square purse over her shoulder that sways with every stride. She notices someone heading across the field toward her but doesn't slow her pace.

He demands her money. She lets her purse slide off her shoulder; the moment it hits the ground, she punches him in the face. Her mood ring smashes into his nose and rips the tender skin beneath it. He lets out a yelp, and then she looks at his face for the first time—he is just a teenager, maybe fifteen. He can't contain all of the blood in his cupped hands. Since her parents are watching her daughter Melissa, she tells him to tilt his head back and to walk. With her fingertips between his shoulder blades, she leans to the side to scoop up her purse and then guides him across the field to her apartment. She tells him to sit down in the kitchen and keep his head tilted. Bright red blood soaks through the towel she has given him to press against the wound. She looks straight at him as she dials the number for the Edmonton police. Dried blood crusted to her fingers cracks as she bends her knuckles. She says into the receiver that someone tried to mug her.

"Where are you now, ma'am?"

"In my apartment."

"Where is he now?"

"In my apartment."

My mom was always really a small-town girl who longed for her backdrops to be quiet landscapes, flat prairies, mostly skies.

My grandparents complained about their eldest daughter living outside the city. Maybe their feelings stemmed from growing up near all of their relatives in Calabria. Or maybe they nurtured an overall disappointment with their rebel daughter who had a baby while unmarried and then later sought a divorce from someone they saw as a "good provider."

"Look here, Jessica," Nanni said while searching through her second kitchen for spare dishes to fill the cupboards of my new apartment. She placed a white mug down on the diner-style table. Her gold wedding band made a ting against its metal surface.

"Your mother's *first* husband gave me this coffee cup." In bold letters the cup read: NUMBER ONE MOTHER-IN-LAW.

Nanni Rose had been promised to a man and didn't go through with it. She must have known what it meant to do what she thought was right despite cultural and family pressures. My grandparents always compared Mom's decisions to her younger brother, Roberto's. *The doctor.* They described his divorce as the fault of his British wife who never learned how to be a *good* wife, because over *there* in England they did things *differently.*

I always thought my parents' decision to raise us in Morinville was part of some lifestyle inheritance, some pull to the rural. The small town, navigated by its residents through landmarks— like Manmade Lake on the town's western edge—and fenced in by wheat and canola fields, is reminiscent of the Calabrian villages where Nanni and Nonno were raised. Something lies at the heart of these small places, some lines run between them. And when I squint into the sunlight, low over the fields, I can almost read them.

When settlers arrived in what would become the village of Morinville, they were attracted to the immensity of the area: wind rushing across the flat ground and a wide sky that offered bright, uninterrupted light. These settlers found clusters of trees, aspen and red spruce, punctuating the prairie, which could offer shade for cattle. In the early days while breaking the first furrows, settlers collected eggs, necessary for survival, that they found in marshy areas and little lakes, giving the name Lac des Oeufs to the area. At this same time, women gave birth to dozens of children. As this parish began to grow, one woman, Mrs. Sara Rondeau, fulfilled the role of midwife no matter the conditions: she waded through snowdrifts as high as her knees and hiked over rough trails to deliver infants.

I try to imagine my hometown in the early twentieth century with just a single street stretching from east to west. The Morinville post office, named after Father Jean-Baptiste Morin, who led the group of early settlers from Quebec, was established in 1892. From that time until 1908, Morinville was considered a village. I see the smooth, paved streets with bright yellow and white lines crumble into loose gravel roadways and the rows of manicured lawns and trim hedges tangle into tall trees. The cul-de-sac where my parent's house now sits is thick with spruce and poplar. I imagine piles of lumber along the roadway. Soon they will be sawed and stuck together to construct the church whose silver steeple will be seen across the flat land. This building, designed by renowned architect J.A. Senecal, will replace the small wooden chapel where residents gather for mass.

Work began on the St. Jean-Baptiste Church mid-summer in 1907, and when it opened its doors on New Years' Day 1908, residents must have been proud of the impressive building with Gothic-style windows and a tower that held the bell donated by Father Morin; the year ahead must have been filled with promise. Each successive priest would contribute to the beauty of the church. By 1912, Father Alexis Gauthier, the fourth priest, had installed stations of the cross, with their benefactors' names inscribed, along the long sidewalls of the church. This building, filled with works by Montreal artists, became known as one of the most beautiful country churches west of Winnipeg. Even now, when people stop in Morinville on their way to somewhere more northern, they comment on the building. *That gorgeous church. What a gorgeous church.*

When I drive down the highway to visit my parents and I see that silver steeple, piercing the prairie sky, I know I am home. When I try to imagine Rosina's St. Antony's Church in Maione, a central part of her life as a devout Catholic, where she carried babies to baptism, a place with resounding bells that echo through all family stories, I picture *that* silver steeple and *those* gravel roads.

Descendants of Morinville's founding families, with French Canadian surnames such as Champagne, Primeau, and Houle, still remain. A large square monument with a cross at the top, which once stood where the roads intersected on Main Street, contains all the founding families' names in small square sections. I have to go to the Church Park to see it now, as it was relocated because it caused too many car accidents. When I run my fingers along the chipped white stone, I recognize every name. As I examine the monument, I wonder about another of Morinville's tributes: the massive, monument-sized toque. This grey and burgundy knit toque was stitched together by more than one hundred volunteers, mostly women from the community. The toque was displayed in the centre of town in the early 1980s and then within the year slipped into some shed where moths and other insects ate through their stitches or made homes in them.

Three of my four siblings have remained in Morinville, and they continue to have Sunday dinners together. Living in a town that encompasses only a few square kilometres enhances this *famiglia* lifestyle in Morinville. It is an echo of a life we might have had in Maione.

Residents and former residents of Maione have formed an online community called The Scattered on a social networking site. After copying and pasting the group's description into an online translator, I learned that it gives second and third generations of emigrants an opportunity to discover their Italian origins and allows family members remaining in Italy to remember those who left. I clicked to a page that listed the members and ran my finger down the screen. Many had the same surnames as my Italian relatives in Edmonton: Pagnotta, Ferrari, and Russo. It didn't take long before a few of us were exchanging family documents and extending the branches of our family trees after we discovered where our roots crossed.

Many people have posted photos. I clicked through shots of people leaning together, standing on cobble streets with backdrops of hills and grainy sunsets. I don't have any photos of my family in Maione, or the other Calabrian villages to contribute to the group. No sunset backdrops or cousins in soccer jerseys. I hesitated for a moment and considered my membership. Then I decided that Rosina, whose photo I now press between the pages of my journal, the top right corner tucked into the book's spine, is not just my matriarch, not just my great-great-grandmother; she is a central part of my family and a central part of the village community. Even if I don't belong in this group, she certainly does.

As I scan the photo, the bright light moves across it, illuminating it from behind. Her long black dress, wrinkles on her hands, and dark eyes stand out against her stark white backdrop, some stucco wall, somewhere in Calabria. And there she is on my computer screen—Rosina.

When I click on the image, I zoom in closer to each line on her face, until the photo is pixilated into a grey blur and I cannot make out her features. I upload the only photo of Rosina to the collective photo album belonging to The Scattered. I write a caption: "Rosina. Her married name is Rosina Russo. 1883–1969. Calabria. Photographer unknown." I press submit. Now this photo, so delicately preserved in Nanni's china cabinet behind those glittery glass doors, after miraculously making its way to Edmonton, is also preserved here, in this fluid new community.

The next morning, as I am leaning against the kitchen counter waiting for the coffee to finish brewing, I remember Rosina on the Internet. I rush to turn on my computer to see if anyone has responded. I feel nervous as I click my way into the group because part of me wants to keep her within the small world of my family. No one has said anything directly about Rosina, but I notice that a new document has been added to the group. It is an unlined sheet of paper with messy printing in blue and black ink. On the centre of the page, the surname *Benincasa* is circled. As far as we know, few official documents exist with Rosina's original family name. Many in the farming villages were illiterate. Those who did read and write often confused the various dialects so even if there are more documents, they may never be located.

When I ask Nanni and Nonno about the Calabrian language, they immediately argue over the phrase "Dear God," which gives me the impression that I have prompted a longstanding dialect debate. Nanni is adamant that it is "O Dio mio," and Nonno is firm that she is wasting her time with the O. I type Altilia and Maione into Google Maps and press the Get Directions button. The thin purple squiggle connecting villages shows that my grandparents grew up only four kilometres apart. The accumulation of slight variances in spelling and pronunciation even between their two villages, in a world where records were kept by pen and paper, suggests fissures in the branches of our family tree, cracks apt to impart tiny splinters.

I flatten a poster-sized family tree of the Ferrari family—my mother's paternal line—on my floor. I pin down the corners with a coffee mug and books. The topmost branches contain the names of four men: my great-grandfather, Sebastiano Santo Ferrari; his father, Francesco Ferrari; his grandfather, Basillo Ferrari; and his great-grandfather, Fernando Ferrari. I watch as these names scatter to the branches below, often as first names, but also sometimes as middle names.

I examine more closely the lines that connect parents to their children and discover that my great-grandfather Sebastiano had six children, one of whom is my Nonno Filippo. All of Sebastiano's children married and had children. Out of the six children, three of them lost their first-borns. All of these babies died before their first birthdays. All were named after Sebastiano's paternal line: baby Santo, baby Francesca, and baby Fernando. The dates startle me: January 31, 1948, to October 26, 1948; March 14, 1950, to November 26, 1950; October 10, 1949, to July 1, 1950. These little lives span less than one year. These years were just prior to emigration.

Perhaps Dr. Iachetta was too far away, or the populations in the villages, now so swollen, meant people had even less access to doctors. I type Dr. Iachetta and Grimaldi and click Search. I find a webpage dedicated to a Dr. Giovanni Iachetta. The direct online translation of the page from Italian to English says that this John Iachetta was born to ancient stock of Grimaldese. Iachetta was tempted to enrol in law school but instead took medicine at the University of Naples, a path assigned to him by God. In addition to regular work, Iachetta also performed some surgeries and dental care. I scroll through the sections that praise his service as a medical officer during the Second World War when he travelled difficult terrain, even at night, to get to patients by the light of his lantern. I notice a section about childbirth. It notes that the war years were a difficult time, especially for the unborn, and states that the "good doctor" was often there along with a midwife. The section notes, in parentheses, that "the midwife is not enough," and then describes the many smiles of joy from pleased mothers thanks to Dr. Iachetta's "tools of the trade . . . forceps . . . and proven ability." He died in 1968, one year before Rosina. Despite all the infants she helped to find their first breath, her skills as a midwife are not mentioned in any type of document, nor honoured in the public record.

Were my sister Melissa's miscarriages something more than "sometimes it just isn't meant to be," or "women lose babies," and caused by some condition passed down in the family? Are these documented losses a part of our genetic inheritance?

Nanni Rose tells me she was relieved that she gave birth to her five children in Edmonton and not in Calabria, although she remembered wishing for Rosina at her side. Her mother, Michelina, like the rest of the women in the village, was instructed to stay in bed for one month after giving birth and was told not to eat any solid food because it could harm her baby.

"Mom would crawl out of bed, weak from not moving for so long, and make dinner. She'd make a chicken for the family and then she would drink the leftover broth. That was it."

"Who told them to do this?" I ask.

"It's just the way it always was. No one person told them. When you heard something, you believed it, or at least you didn't tempt fate. Women were afraid they would lose their babies, so they did what their mothers and Nannis did. And prayed."

After reading the names and dates of these Ferrari babies, I can better understand why Nanni and Nonno instructed my mother to pin a cloth packet of salt to Melissa when she was an infant. Nanni pulls out a tissue and folds it into a square to demonstrate. First, she would place the red cloth down on the counter and fill it with salt. Then she would press a small figurine of St. Antony down in the middle. Then with a threaded needle, she'd stitch the cloth into a square. It was sewn tightly and rolled between the finger and thumb to make sure none of the salt fell out. Nanni shakes the bunched-up tissue and then places it against her black T-shirt.

"See? Like this."

Melissa, my mom's first-born and also my grandparents' first grandchild, wore this red cloth packet safety-pinned to her clothes whenever she left the house. When she was a little older, she had a small red ribbon sewn into the seam of her clothing. It was believed by some in Calabria that this red package and ribbon protected the baby from the evil eye. This ribbon was a preventative measure against severe infant illness or even death caused by this evil force. The red ribbon wasn't the only superstitious practice in the villages. If villagers walked beneath the branches of a walnut tree after dark with a baby in their arms, or in a sling across them, it was believed the baby would soon die. The only way to thwart this death was to chop off a branch; many people avoided any routes lined with walnut trees, a difficult task in a rural farming village where trees bordered crops to shield them from the wind.

"You saw a lot of branchless trees. Just a tall trunk sticking out of the ground," Nonno explains as he points upwards.

A maternal tree that includes Rosina has been clear-cut over time. It's difficult to trace the lines of women when no one has kept clear records and husbands' last names replace women's first family surnames. What of Rosina's mother? Her grandmother? Her great-grandmother? What were their names? I think of these women every time my stomach spins as I look at the blurry world through a car window. I know that the motion sickness in my mother's family trickles down through the women, but with whom did it begin? What was her name? These women could be snapped off the tree like the walnut branches, and soon no one would know they had existed.

I can't read a word on the scanned image of the sheet with Benincasa circled in the centre, except for the names: Geniale Benincasa, Antonia Porco, Michele Benincasa, and Rosina Benincasa. Still I feel hopeful that I may have discovered some of the names surrounding Rosina's. Are these her relatives? Parents? Siblings? When I paste the words into an online translator and select Italian to English, nothing comes out right except for the caption added to the document: "Can someone translate this for Jessica?"

I send Romano, the man who added the document to The Scattered, an email that says, "Grazie! Grazie!" though I feel embarrassed for not understanding Italian. I wait a few more days. I wonder if I should print out the document and take it to my grandparents for some translation help; though, with their dialogue debates and Nanni's poor eyesight, I decide to wait. Instead, I click through the new photos.

I stop on a striking landscape posted by a woman named Maria. The caption on the photo reads: "The beautiful little town where I was born." The town, cozy between deep green hills, is Maione. I find myself tracing its shape, a near oval from the angle of the shot, and I wonder which orange-roofed homes belonged to my relatives. Is one of these homes on land where Rosina lived with her parents? When I click Maria's name, I discover that she now lives in Toronto, Ontario. Maria's family likely emigrated in the 1950s, when so many Calabrians established a community in central Canada.

Toronto's Italian community often meets at the restaurants and businesses along College Street West, stopping in at Bitondos for pizza or hanging out at the Sicilian Ice Cream shop; this is one of the largest Canadian gatherings in the diaspora. The 2006 census documented that Ontario's Italian Canadian population was 865,000, more than double the size of the community in any other province: Italian immigrants scattered to central Canada like fennel seeds through fingers.

❧   ❧   ❧

I signalled my turn off the Yellowhead Trail in north Edmonton. I curved away from the heavy traffic and cement walls and drove down 97th Street, with the city's gapped skyline as my backdrop. When I spotted the bright red BENVENUTI sign arched over 95th Street, I slowed down to find a place to park.

As I sipped my latte at Spinelli's Bar Italia in Edmonton's Little Italy, I wondered why so many emigrants made their way west and rerooted their families in the prairies. It doesn't surprise me that most records didn't make the journey across the ocean in the suitcases that contained households. I imagine histories like leaves, scattering on sea breezes and on those cool whispers that rustle the trees. And names, those little specks that make sunsets grainy.

On a Thursday morning in 2010, the small café attached to the Italian Centre Shop was busier than I had expected. Most tables were filled with men drinking lattes while others leaned against the bar sipping espressos and reaching into the tall jars of biscotti. A couple stood at the bar waiting to purchase pastries and went over their grocery list, reciting what they needed to buy, half in Italian and half in English.

In the corner of the café was a large painting of a southern Italy washed in orange light. The landscape is likely San Pietro al Tanagro of Campania, the hometown of Frank Spinelli, the southern Italian who opened the shop in 1959 after immigrating to Edmonton.

The walls, lined with shelves of framed Italia soccer photos, soccer plaques, and red and green soccer balls, boast of Italian pride. Across from me, an old man slouched in a chair with his legs crossed at the ankles. His cane rested against the table. He picked at a chocolate-covered croissant and sipped a coffee with swirls of white cream peaking over the rim. Had that been his spot for years? He stared out the window, perhaps daydreaming about Old Italia. He interrupted my romantic imaginings when he reached into his jacket and flipped open his cellphone. He typed a message into the tiny keypad with surprisingly nimble fingers.

N O V E

"You don't look Italian," Teresa Spinelli says. She's asked one of the women behind the counter for a coffee before she sits down beside me.

Or sound like it. Or cook like it. I shrug and smile.

"I'm half Italian, my mom's side."

Teresa leans back in her chair with her hands wrapped around her mug, and I feel like I am at her kitchen table. She greets the customers seated throughout the café, sometimes with a nod that shakes her brunette hair and sometimes with their first names.

"You're a popular woman, Teresa."

"Ah, yeah, well I practically grew up here. I took my first steps over there in the pasta aisle. The customers treat me like family. Some of the older ones have watched me grow up."

I imagine Teresa, now in her late forties, as a baby with round eyes and dark hair waddling past the linguine and tortellini and reaching for the colourful packages. "And now, the next generation watches my son toddle around."

From where I sit in the café, near the entrance to the grocery shop, I can see customers wheeling their red baskets through the aisles, plunking down cans of olives and lupine beans. The café as an extension of the grocery store makes sense. In the 1960s Teresa's father, Frank, rented an old theatre to show Italian films and bring the community together. A statue of Frank Spinelli sits at the edge of Little Italy in Giovanni Caboto Park, just across the street from the shop. The bronze figure wears a shirt, tie, and a heavy leather jacket. He holds a handful of cards. Frank played poker with other Italians at the back of his shop, where they would also share meals, exchange news of home, and plan cultural events in the city.

In 1951, Frank Spinelli arrived near Mayo, Yukon, just in time for the first snowfall of the year. I imagine that in his letters home he wrote of a world of snow and ice: a place where the wind freezes cheeks rather than coats them with dust and sand. He worked in the silver mine alongside other immigrants, chipping into mineral resources that would enrich Canada's expanding economy. In 1954, he broke his back on the worksite.

Frank spent eighteen months in traction in a hospital in Edmonton. While confined, he chatted with nurses and other patients—learning new words for familiar things and new sounds for others that he had never known before. *La Spina*. Back. *Dolore*. Pain. After he was discharged, he and other Italian men drove Edmonton's streets in his Ford truck in search of work. Frank had loaned much of his compensation money to other Italian immigrants—for mortgages and food.

In 1959, Frank partnered with a friend to open a small shop. Like other corner stores, they stocked items like chocolate bars and pop, but what drew in most of their customers were the imported Italian newspapers and magazines. Soon, their Italian customers complained that they liked reading the news from home in their own language, but that they didn't have any espressos or lattes to drink while they read it. After Frank imported machines and the beans to make lattes and espressos, they asked for pastas. They missed their nanni's spaghetti and mother's soup with fresh bread, the foods they grew up with. In the early years of Frank's business, his customers were almost all Italian.

A year after the small shop was established, Frank married Rina Quagliarello, a woman from his village. Frank's mother chose Rina as his wife and their marriage took place by proxy. It was not long before Rina left her family in San Pietro al Tanagro to join Frank in Edmonton.

The story goes that after a year or so of living in Edmonton, Rina was about to give birth to their first child. At that same time, my Nanni Rose was in the same hospital, on the same floor, giving birth to her third baby. Rina was in a lot of pain and cried out, but the nurses didn't know what she was saying. A nurse asked Rose to go and talk to her, to see if she could comfort her and stop the wailing. Just before Rose entered Rina's room, a family member or neighbour arrived and she was no longer needed. However, the first time I heard the story, Nanni Rose entered Rina's room, spoke with her, and offered words of comfort. Either way, Teresa Spinelli and my uncle Giuliano Ferrari were born just a few days apart that October in 1961.

Frank had taken over the shop by 1964 and needed a larger space. He was turned down for a bank loan and had to obtain one through a finance company that charged high interest rates. Frank employed Peter Batoni's construction company to build his new shop—soon to be the largest business in Little Italy. By this time, more than fifteen thousand Italian Canadians lived in Alberta, and many lived in Edmonton.

Frank worked with two Italians living in Calgary, Tony Falcone and Alberto Romano, in a campaign to legalize home wine making. In Italy, people had been making wine and clinking their glasses together at their kitchen tables for generations, but when they arrived in Canada in the 1950s they realized this practice was illegal. The province of Alberta had a long history of banning alcohol, and making wine at home was still forbidden.

The law could be traced to 1915, when Alberta's all-male electorate voted the province as dry as Drumheller. Sixty-one percent favoured Prohibition. The law was enacted on Canada Day 1916: all liquor stores and bars would be closed and no liquor would be sold in the province. The coal mining towns of the Crowsnest Pass, full of European immigrants, as well as small communities such as St. Albert and Morinville, populated largely by French Canadians, voted wet, but the drys outnumbered them. In *The Rum Runners*, stories of Prohibition in Canada, Frank Anderson writes that even in 1917 Alberta was still quite damp as large amounts of alcohol were smuggled across the provincial border in trunks and suitcases. By 1918, the federal government had tightened regulations. Liquor traffic went underground and evolved into rum running, an industry with a connection to some early Italian immigrants—a history later immortalized in the Canadian opera *Filumena*.

Sicilian-born Emilio Picariello, owner of the Alberta Hotel in Blairmore in the Crowsnest Pass, became known as Emperor Pic, a huge personality on the Prohibition scene in Alberta. He was a man who kept a wolf on a chain and stored thousands of dollars in the floorboards of his truck. Business-minded Emilio saw the potential of smuggling liquor. He poured cement into the metal bumpers of his trucks to enable them to smash through barriers. He loaded up his Fords with sacks of flour and stashed burlap bags of alcohol among them and when he returned from running trips, the sacks of unused flour were given to families in the area.

One story tells of a rainy night when Picariello's vehicle became stuck. His tires barely turned in the thick muck. He walked along the roadway until he came upon a lit farmhouse. Inside, two police constables, trying to stay dry, were watching their road through the window, scanning for rum runners. The constables helped heave Picariello's car free, rocking it back and forth until it finally pulled forward. They wished the farmer dressed in soaked overalls good luck on his travels and Emperor Pic drove away. I see him flinging his hand up to the sky in a sardonic gesture of thanks as he looked back at them in his rear-view mirror.

In the early fall of 1922, a constable in Blairmore received a tip about a liquor delivery. Steve Picariello, Emilio's nineteen-year-old son, was one of the runners on this particular trip and he was heading toward his father's Blairmore hotel. A high-speed car chase began. Steve sped off toward the British Columbia border, but before he crossed the provincial line he was shot by Constable Lawson, who had stepped out in the street, hand outstretched before his chest, feet apart, and ready to negotiate. The constable later reported that Steve did not show any signs of slowing down, and that he had to jump out of the way of the speeding vehicle. Constable Lawson pulled the trigger. With a bullet wound in his hand, Steve sped off. Emilio heard about the shooting and, unaware of the extent of his son's injuries and assuming the worst, decided to confront Lawson.

Filumena Lassandro, known as Florence after she immigrated to Alberta from southern Italy, had, at age fourteen, married one of Emilio Picariello's close associates, a man who was ten years older than her. Her husband worked for Emilio, and while she regularly completed the housekeeping and watched over Emilio's children, she was also often persuaded to go along with his son Steve on rum-running trips as the police would likely not suspect this young couple of illegal activity.

After the shooting, Filumena accompanied Emilio on a frantic drive to find Constable Lawson. Lassandro later testified that Picariello, upon finding Lawson, said to him, "You shot my boy and you're going with me to get him." Lawson stated that he didn't know where Emilio's son was.

The young woman watched the argument from the passenger seat. Picariello pulled out his gun to force the constable to come with them to find his son, and the two struggled until the gun was fired several times—one shot went through the windshield. When Lassandro looked over, she saw that Picariello was struggling to breathe. The constable had his arms around her friend's neck. She fired at the constable, and he released his grip.

Lawson fell backwards from the blow and died on the pavement. I imagine tiny crystals of glass all over Filumena's lap as the two sped away. In 1923, Filumena Lassandro was hanged next to Emilio Picariello at the Fort Saskatchewan jail—the last woman to be executed in Alberta.

By 1964, Frank and other advocates had successfully lobbied to change the law to allow the making of wine at home. Soon after wine making was permitted, Frank became the biggest grape supplier in Edmonton. Some years he had upwards of forty thousand cases of dark grapes in wooden crates stacked in his warehouse and his shop.

Nonno taught my dad the art of Italian wine making. Long before the deep red liquid fermented, they would drink the *grappa* after dinner, always commenting on just how *good* the *bad* wine was. Mom would remind Dad that he had to drive home.

"Ah, no! Just stay over!" Nonno would say as they clinked their glasses together.

"I'll make a big breakfast in the morning. Fatten the kids up," Nanni would say as she put her arm around my shoulders. I thought it was good that Nonno and Dad got along, even as the night wore on and they kept splashing wine into their glasses. I remembered hearing a story about Nonno and some threat. Some big argument on Mom and Dad's doorstep in Morinville. I always pretended that it was a movie they had been talking about, but as I got older, it seemed more likely: a new man just after a divorce. A new man with long, blond curly hair, a man from the country. Maybe when Mom announced that she was pregnant with me, just one year before they married, her parents gave up trying to stop the relationship, let her trespass the borderlines they would never remove.

Dad inherited wine lessons and he listened to stories of grape growing from the Old Country while they discarded stems and debris and swished around liquids. The final product, a long-fermented unlabelled bottle of red wine, became a passport necessary to cross the borders Nonno had created. Nonno would inspect the wine in the big glass bottle and say, "See. See. Look at that! It's good! Yeah?"

Nonno stored huge jugs in his wine shed, a temperature-controlled room that he made himself. We would drive to Nanni's and Nonno's place to help squish grapes through rollers, separating the juice from the dark skin. I'd press a purple ball between my thumb and forefinger; the skin was soft and the insides ready to burst. I'd roll it back and forth until the skin let go and the translucent insides popped onto the floor. As I piled the stems into wooden crates, Mom would watch and talk about how there was no roller when she was young; instead, she had to hide her purple feet in socks.

Once Dad had practised the skills, he started to make his own wine, filling the shelves of our basement storage room with round jars so large that I couldn't stretch my arms around them. When I twisted off the black caps, the smell rushed up my nose and throat, a fiery smell that reminded me of secrets. It burned my nostrils and tongue. I twisted the cap back on. *Grappa. Grappa. Grappa.*

     ❧   ❧   ❧

Teresa Spinelli is president of the Italian Centre Shop, a role she inherited when her father, Frank, died suddenly in 2000. Although she was the eldest child, the shop was meant to go to her younger brother, Pietro. In a traditional Italian family, that was the way it was, but Pietro died shortly after his thirty-second birthday.

Teresa has opened a second location outside Little Italy on the south side of Edmonton, a shop that boasts a more upscale location. Both stores feature sections of foods from other countries: Poland, Cuba, Germany. Teresa explains that before Polish immigrants came to Canada, many lived in Italy first for two or three years. They came into the Italian Centre Shop looking for the foods they had enjoyed in this interim period but then started requesting that Teresa import specialties like the chocolates and soups that reminded them of their Polish grandmothers.

"Once, a Cuban man called the shop and asked for me. He wanted to thank me for hiring his son. He explained that he immigrated here with nothing and was really grateful."

"What about your other employees. Are they mostly Italian?" I ask as I glance behind the counter at the woman with long brown hair and perfect black eyeliner.

"Many of them are. It's funny because some of the younger women that work here, their parents never went back to Italy. They came in hard times and that's the image they have of it."

Teresa, who has been travelling back and forth since she was five, shakes her head and drops her hands to the table. "They live by those old traditions. Their daughters can't go out. They have early curfews. Their mentality stayed the same. And when they say, 'That's how it is in Italy, where we are from' they are not speaking about Italy now."

"So, the place stayed fixed," I say, realizing that Nanni Rose's version of Italy remained unchanged in her mind, peopled by those long gone.

"Yeah, exactly. But, in some ways, even those traditions affect me. I feel like I have to cook, even though my husband does not care, he says not to. I'm busy, but I feel like I should."

Teresa came into her role as president without preparation.

She had gone to university rather than study the way the shop was run, and she had expected her brother to assume her father's position. Once she mastered the business basics, she started to do things her own way, and before long, the shop was booming.

"You know, I only became a mother a few years ago, when I was forty-five. My mother had two children by the age of twenty-four and I wasn't even married until I was thirty-seven when I then found out I couldn't have children," Teresa says. She tucks her hair behind her ear, leans in closer to the table.

She flattens her palms on the table and tells me that years earlier, she and her husband had tried adoption. Eventually she pulled her name off the adoption list, sure that it wasn't going to happen. She and her husband took expensive cooking classes and did a lot of travelling. They built a fine home, one without a spare bedroom, and were busy with the business. Then, one day a few years ago, a pregnant woman came into the shop. Her round belly signalled that she was quite far along. Teresa learned that she was only two weeks from her due date. The woman wanted Teresa to adopt her baby.

"How did she know you?"

"I guess through my work in the community," Teresa explained. "At first I thought, no, there is no way. That idea was long behind us. We hadn't considered it for years. But then I went home and told my husband. We slept on it. Did a lot of crying and praying. The next day, we knew he was ours."

"Do you speak Italian to Massimo?" I ask.

"Yes and other people here do too when I bring him to the shop."

"Is he Italian?" I ask. My stomach turns the second the words take shape, because the answer doesn't matter. He was more Italian than I'd ever be.

❧ ❧ ❧

I hadn't expected Nanni and Nonno to know much about the Spinelli family. They knew the village they were from and told me the story about Frank's success in Edmonton. In that moment, I saw Edmonton not as a sprawling city but as a reflection of the tiny village that they had left behind. I saw the lines of streets overlap and curve.

When Nonno pointed outside their front bay window and told me how dangerous Edmonton had become, I watched the city spread out again: concrete buildings thrust upwards on the flat ground, a grid of streets and bumpy back alleyways. Nanni warned me not to get involved with the *wrong* people because that's *all* it takes for life to go awry; I wondered if this fear kept Nanni and Nonno in the same area in North Edmonton, and if this fear is what kept the Italian community together. Nonno leaned forward and while blinking through his thick dark lashes and scratching the top of his head said, "Yep. That's *all* it takes. And it's even harder for immigrants to build a good life, with so much already against them."

"There's other things out there too," Nanni added.

"What other things?"

"Some people have had hard lives, and it makes them . . . a little . . . I don't know . . . crazy," Nanni said and then straightened the coasters on the table.

"Who are you talking about, Nan?" She shrugged, as if the story was over before it started. "Who?" I asked again.

"She was raised by the nuns."

"Someone in Edmonton?"

"Her dad remarried right after his wife died. She didn't go to school or anything, they just kept her there for a time."

"Who?" I asked as I turned to Nonno, since it was clear Nanni was trying to keep a secret stitched together.

"The lady, whose mother died in Calabria a long, long time ago. She went to live with the nuns. The nuns raised the baby girl. They kept her there. She didn't go to school or anything. There are sad things in the world. Hard things."

"Where is she now?" I asked Nonno.

"In Edmonton. She emigrated," he answered while looking at Nanni.

"What's her name?"

"Ah," Nanni started, "I don't remember."

I nodded, and all I could think was *grappa, grappa, grappa*. I imagined secrets swishing around the burgundy-stained glass. I felt like *this* secret was a serious one, and I knew I couldn't ask any more questions.

D I E C I

overlay a translucent print placed over a map
detailing something not visible on the original

A few days after I posted Rosina's photo online, the translation
arrived from The Scattered:

> Around 1870 in Altilia/Maione there existed only
> one family with the name Benincasa. Benincasa
> is a very common name especially in the town of
> Mangone. In 1895/96 the office of records for mili-
> tary service confirms Michele Benincasa born in
> Altilia-Maione 17-9-1876 son of Geniale Benincasa
> and Antonia Porco. It is very probable that Rosina
> is the sister of that Michele.

If there is only one registered family in Altilia and Maione with the Benincasa surname, then *this* is likely *them*—Rosina's brother, Michele, her father, Geniale, and her mother, Antonia. War leaves records. It is striking that there was only one Benincasa family registered in these villages because homes and land often remained in families for generations. Maybe the Benincasas, Geniale's ancestors, were from Mangone, the hilly village just northeast of Altilia and Maione, but he was offered a deal on some land and so moved his family down the river to Altilia. Perhaps they returned on Sundays to Mangone to visit their relatives and bring them some ripe produce or a sack of wheat.

Maybe Michele, strong from years of working in the field behind Geniale, would offer to carry the sack over one shoulder. The wheat, pressed firm against his back, would move with every stride, sometimes spilling out the top and scattering on the dry ground, leaving a trail between villages. Sometimes Antonia and Rosina would stay behind, collecting tomatoes that grew up the side of the house, fruit so soft under the heat it was easy to press a finger through. The warm seeds would ooze through the elastic red skin.

Or, maybe they didn't work at all, and instead they sat inside the cool corners of the house and talked about the men who left for America and came back with little to show for it. Maybe they pulled the cork from a jug of wine taken from the cellar, a sweet snap against the glass, took a drink and then swished water around in their mouths and rubbed away the dark evidence from their lips.

Maybe Antonia never wanted children, and so ignored her daughter, and they just worked, wordlessly, side by side, sweating in their thick cotton dresses as they squeezed and scrubbed the household's clothes. And when Antonia bent over the river to rinse off the soap, she'd catch a glimpse of her face on the rippling surface of the water. When she saw herself, she'd imagine her body wrapped in the silks she had seen in the shop window in Mangone, clothing so smooth that it would feel like a wave against her skin, especially when the wind went through it. But maybe Antonia wasn't Rosina's mother, or even her aunt or relation at all. Maybe *these* Benincasas are not *them*. In my mind Antonia unravels and disappears—smooth blue silk on the riverbank.

With a pencilled line, I attach mother to daughter on the matriarchal tree. *Antonia—Rosina.* I imagine that if she were her mother, she taught Rosina to boil acorns until they were tender. Antonia would have passed on her knowledge about pregnancy and childbirth, maybe even told Rosina about her own labour stories or the deliveries of other women she knew. She was probably the one to teach her about holy water and suction. Last rites and evil eyes. And about stitching everything together when it pulled apart.

When I calculate the dates, the story fits. Michele, seven years older than Rosina, was her big brother. Perhaps 1895 was Michele's first year of military service, and he went to fight in Ethiopia the following year in Battle of Adwa, the first Italo-Abyssinian War. If Michele had not yet been married and still lived with his parents, this would have been the last time these siblings lived under the same roof. Rosina was married the next year, and would become known as Rosina Russo, Giovanni's wife, even if her name remained unchanged in the records. Women often left their own families and moved into the houses their husbands shared with their parents. I imagine Rosina's girlhood slip into the river and travel downstream along with the laundry bubbles.

I've never heard any stories about young Rosina or about her parents and siblings. All of the stories start with her marriage to Giovanni at fifteen, when she became Rosina Russo. The new surname, while it may not have been changed in official records, stitched itself to her, identified her as *his* wife, as *his* children's mother. Nanni Rose usually tells me about her beloved Rosina in these roles. Other stories refer to her position as a midwife, the woman who stepped in when *Dottor* Iachetta couldn't be there. The rest are about how hard it was for everyone to leave her behind.

I follow fictional lines until I've fashioned an entire extended family. I house them. I watch their fields grow. Rosina is alive within those lines, no matter how limiting they can be.

❧   ❧   ❧

Some coloured funeral cards scatter to the table as Nanni shakes the papers out of the white plastic bag. Several typewritten pages with circular seals and square stamps land around our teacups and bowls of grapes. Most of the words are so faded that, even if I could read Italian, I wouldn't be able to make them out. I reach for three funeral cards tucked inside of one another, all for women, all in black and white. Each woman's hair is pulled back, and not one is smiling in the glossy photo on the front. The photographs selected for the cards seem to reflect the mourners' feelings, not capture the personality of the deceased. Each card includes each woman's name, birth date, death date, and a short religious poem. *L'onesta fu il suo ideale. Il lavoro la sua vita. La famiglia il suo affetto.* Honesty was his ideal, work was his life, family his affection.

These women were three of Rosina's daughters. There is no card for the fourth, and Nanni Rose cannot remember this aunt's name or her place in the birth order. I pick up the card of Teresina, the oldest of these three daughters, and subtract the year Teresina was born, 1899, from the year that Rosina was born. Rosina was sixteen when her daughter Teresina arrived.

Another paper offers scant details about a woman named Anna. The dashes between her dates tell me that she was born just a few years after Rosina in 1887 and died a few years before Rosina in 1966. Nanni shrugs when I ask about her about Anna and continues to flip through the other papers. She finds a small photo of this woman. Her wrinkled neck is loose and her eyebrows droop over the corner of her eyes. Her nose seems to spread flat across her face, and her smile, so slight, is contagious, as if she is about to break into a laugh. Was she part of the Benincasa family, a name to add as a sibling to Michele and Rosina? A cousin? Or did she marry into the family? An in-law?

I realize how traceable we have become in our own era. So many of our records would survive a fire or an international move and will be preserved through time. I have three email accounts, two professional and one personal. Each is stuffed with records of friendships, receipts from online purchases, grades, and resumés. I keep lengthy emails from my mom and brother and even notes and reminders that I have sent to myself. These virtual records—I imagine them as blasts of coloured energy—in that *other* life, *online*—can be retrieved in an instant. Typed words can be copied and pasted and put into online translators that will spit out a variation of the intended meaning and, even if not entirely accurate, can be read in any language.

Nanni runs her hands over the papers on the table and picks up a few. She squints at the words. Nonno drags his slippered feet across the tiled floor into the kitchen and slides in next to her. They both bend over the pages, sounding out the faded Italian.

"My family was going to throw these out when we cleaned out Mom and Dad's house. I can't believe that. They had saved them for all that time. They weren't garbage. So I kept them," Nanni explains with her hands near her face and her shoulders hunched.

By the time Nanni Rose and her siblings sorted through their parents' things, her oldest brother, Giovanni, was gone. He died in the summer of 1994 of a heart attack, just like his Nonno Giovanni—his namesake. And just like Rosina, his wife, Lena, found him. They had been out at Half Moon Lake. Giovanni was piling bricks to make a fireplace when it happened; he was airlifted to a hospital in Edmonton. The autopsy report showed that his arteries were blocked, and through tests, doctors determined that it was a genetic problem. I remember that was the summer we were in British Columbia camping, and Nanni called Mom at the campground. A message was left at the campground's office for Mom to call her mother right away. I sat at a picnic table and heard Mom repeat the news into the payphone's receiver. "He is dead. A heart attack. Oh, God, no!"

I wondered if Lena thought of Rosina *Vecchia*, her grand-mother-in-law, sometime after her husband was gone. Rosina, the woman left behind in Italy and in the field that day so many years before, and now Lena, left behind at the lake.

Once Giovanni died, Nanni Rose, the second-born, inherited the role as the keeper of family documents, secrets, and stories. Nanni keeps a shard of a small, once-square mirror wrapped in a piece of brown paper. When I hold it, the pointed tip fits in my palm between my thumb and forefinger. This is what remains of Nanni Rose's first mirror, which she used to see her reflection clearly for the first time. Before that, she had tried to glimpse herself in tarnished spoons, a metal bucket, and on the surface of the river. The mirror was a gift from her big brother, Giovanni; he gave it to her when they were reunited in Edmonton.

Nonno nods as he pulls his finger across the top of a page while reading the words out loud. Comune Di Altilia. I peer over his shoulder and see a chart. Benincasa Rosina is typed across the bottom row.

"Nonno, what is this?"

"An inventory."

Most of the papers that I pick up are in Italian, and I ask if I can make copies so that I can pore over them with my English–Italian dictionary, but Nanni starts to tuck them all back into the bag. I look at the sheet that Nonno has just picked up.

"A copy of my immigration approval," he says, flicking the sheet upwards and flashing it at me. The original was handed over when he arrived in Halifax.

"I came alone. All by myself."

✿   ✿   ✿

Nanni and Nonno explain that before they could leave Italy, southern residents travelled to Rome, where they would undergo medical examinations and obtain passports. Nanni Rose's cousin, Francesco Barona, was her bridge into this new world of documentation and verification, of exchanging money for signatures and stamps. On the second page of her passport, written in jagged cursive, is the strange word that came clumsily off her tongue: *Canada*.

Francesco walked back into the village after seven years away. In his absence, the shift had already started to happen: men were leaving. Francesco had fought in the Second World War and became a prisoner of the English sometime before it ended. He was kept on a farm. Nonno explains that the English kept him there against his will, but Nanni says the English were kind and saved his life, offering a place to hide from the Germans who would have shot him.

"He was in trouble for something. Something was wrong and he needed protection," Nanni explains. "He worked on the English farm in exchange for food and somewhere to sleep."

Francesco's mother, that Teresina on the funeral card, thought he was dead and would lie awake at night crying for her son. Her sobs became a part of the daily rhythm of the house, her grief as predictable as day falling into night.

"My aunt Teresina cried for years. But Rosina, her mom, told her not to worry because he was alive. She knew. Even when the war was officially over and he was still gone, Rosina told her that it was early yet, he'd come home."

Sometime in 1946, Teresina was out in the yard and looked toward the road. She spotted a figure in the distance, walking home.

As I pick up her funeral card, I imagine that still woman with the smooth face and small dark eyes bunch her skirt up to her knees and run toward her son, "Dio mio! Francesco!" As they pull along the coast, Rose tells her cousin the tale of his return, as if he wasn't a part of it but a character in a story.

***

On the train to Rome, Francesco told his younger cousin Rose and her brother Vittorio stories about the war and about England. He explained that there had not been any water to drink. He'd wait until it rained and the water collected in the horseshoe prints on the ground. He'd bend down, cheek to the ground, and slurp the few centimetres of water that had collected in the hoof print. Rose told him that all of his mother's tears could have slaked his thirst.

"You came right over to our place, because you wanted to see Nanni Rosina. She knew you were alive. She didn't look surprised to see you but just held her hands against your face and smiled. Your mom was pale as a ghost. She stared at you without blinking. And you needed a haircut."

Francesco told them of the world beyond Italy. Rose admitted she was scared that she wouldn't pass her medical examination and be able to go and see her dad. She had heard stories about people who were denied their documents. Without those papers, she worried that everyone would leave and she'd be forgotten.

When she arrived in the office, she saw women standing in a line that started at the back of the room and curved around all four walls. A doctor made his way through them, while writing notes on his clipboard. Some women, frail in old age, leaned on their sisters or daughters. Some women held babies they shushed as they swayed back and forth.

The doctor handed her the crisp sheet of paper with his inky signature in the corner. Rose passed the test. She rushed to show Francesco and Vittorio, who were waiting on a bench outside. Vittorio clutched his bright white papers and Rose waved hers at him. Francesco got up and put his arm around her but didn't act as happy as she had expected. They three walked together to their hotel; the coins that Michelina had given Francesco to pay for the room clinked in his pocket. The next morning, Rose and Vittorio would get their passports.

A year before Rose's trip to Rome with Francesco, Filippo Ferrari had made the same trip. He was asked to strip naked in a roomful of other men. Beneath the bright lights, he felt small in his body. After a childhood of chronic illness and trips to see Dr. Iachetta, he was sure he wouldn't pass the examination.

Next to him, a man with thick muscles argued with the doctor, told him about his family already in Toronto waiting for him. The doctor just shook his head and pointed toward the door. Filippo had heard that some women and men paid healthier people to pass the medical test for them. After they had the papers, they would walk to the passport office and get their own photo taken. It was risky, but those who wanted to leave had made up their minds, and most of those who wanted to stay needed the money.

Just before the doctor asked his name, Filippo looked down at his bony knees and tried to push up his chest. The doctor decided Filippo was healthy. He arrived in Canada less than a year later, in February 1954. Rose and Vittorio followed in May 1955.

More than twenty years later, Filippo and Rose were driving through Clareview in northeast Edmonton to get some groceries at Superstore when he admitted to his wife that he felt sick. Rose told him that he had to stop being stubborn and just go to see their family doctor.

The doctor listened to his chest, tested his reflexes, and then stood back and said, "Mr. Ferrari, your skin appears yellow."

Filippo leaned over to look at his reflection in the clinic's mirror. His face did look a bit off, but he just shrugged.

"Ah, Doctor. It's just the lighting."

The doctor sent him for tests and reminded him that no news

is good news. A few days later, Rose, busy getting dinner on the table, shook off her oven mitt and answered the phone. Filippo had to go back to the clinic the next morning.

"But I have to work!" he said and threw his hands up in the air. "I'm feeling fine."

"You won't be able to work if you're dead! You're going! First thing in the morning!"

When Filippo arrived at the clinic, he was sent right in to see the doctor. The doctor pulled his stool near Filippo's chair and with his hands on his lap said, "Mr. Ferrari, you have tuberculosis. You've had it for a number of years, probably since you were a child. Did you live on a farm?"

"Yes."

"Did you handle any goats or lambs in Italy?"

"Yes."

"Mr. Ferrari, did you ever drink right from a cow's nipple?" he asked, while pinching his fingers open and closed.

"Oh, yes. When I got thirsty. We all did."

"Ah, well, that is likely how you got it. I'm surprised they never caught that when you emigrated. You wouldn't have been cleared to leave."

I've seen copies of both Nanni and Nonno's passports. My brother Jason made photocopies when he applied for dual citizenship, and he asked if I wanted to see them. In Nonno's, his thick dark hair is piled tall on his head. It looks like it has been styled to stand straight. He is wearing a plaid button-up shirt and a dark jacket. His collar is tucked in. His head is angled to the right. His face is smooth as stone, and his eyebrows are thick black arches.

The page opposite his photo reads: *Repubblica Italiana. 1953. Il Ministero degli Affari Esteri rilascia il presente passaport a Signor FERRARI.*

The passport wasn't made for women. On the calligraphic *Signor* of Nanni's passport, the issuing authority has inked the letters *-ina* to the end of the word.

Nanni's passport photo is eye-catching. She looks like a model, with thick lips and dark lashes. Her black hair is smoothed and pinned back and her blouse is pressed flat. She looks at least twenty years old, though she was only sixteen and would soon be placed in third grade because she didn't know a word of English. She'll be too large for the desk and too ashamed to go to school without any shoes. She'll drop out and sweep a bar for money. Two years later, she will give birth to my mother. The last page before the stamps reads: Destination *EDMONTON*, Occupation *HOUSEKEEPER*.

❧ ❧ ❧

Words typewritten onto official records, shaky signatures, and faded stamps reduce lives to isolated facts and reveal another kind of truth.

Nanni puts the plastic bag of family documents away and tells me I can come and look at them again. Then, after I mention them to my uncle Roberto and he tells his parents that he's interested in them, they give them to him to take home. When Roberto hands me the copies, he laughs and says that there is an order to things.

I spread out all the pages and scan for the inventory, and there it is, a copy, crooked on the page. *Situazione di Famiglia del Sig. Russo Generoso fu Giovanni.* Just above a row of equal signs across the bottom of the page, like a long parallel line, it reads N. 8 Benincasa Rosina.

It is an inventory of the eight people who lived in the house on the hill, until they left, in stages, and Rosina was the only one who remained. Next to the column of names is a column titled *Paternità* and the next, *Maternità*. Next to Rosina's name it reads: Geniale. I can't believe it. The explanation of the registered Benincasa family from The Scattered checks out and I picture Geniale and his son, Michele, walking to Mangone with wheat sacks over their shoulders and Antonia at home uncorking the wine in the cellar. Then my imagination is interrupted as I scan the next column. Next to Geniale, where it should read Antonia, it says: Carmina Pucci.

Next to that pile of blue silk rests a crumpled military uniform.
The final two rows next to Rosina's name read:

Professione: Contadino. Peasant.

Osservazioni: Vedova. Widow.

U N D I C I

I'm certain now that at least two photos exist.

The second one is tucked behind pink and yellow fabric flowers. The bouquet, colourful blooms that will never need watering, spills out of a thin wooden vase and covers most of her face.

The night before we arrived in Calabria, I barely slept. Out of the hotel window in Rome, the sun—a perfect orange circle—glowed like a streetlight through a rain-spotted windshield. I had been asleep for a little more than two hours. The hotel clock read 1:00 AM. I pulled my glasses off the nightstand and slid them on to make sure. When I woke up again, I squinted at the fuzzy red light. The clock read 1:12 AM. Then 1:45 AM. 3:15 AM. 4:03 AM. While in and out of sleep, I kept trying to calculate the eight-hour time difference: the time that it *is* versus the time that it *feels* like. I could not make sense of the Italian sun in the sky during the Italian nighttime. This went on all night, but the sun didn't move. It stayed firmly in the frame of the hotel's square window.

I hadn't slept on the flights from Edmonton to Montreal or Montreal to Rome. My anxiety about searching for traces of a woman I wanted to wholly know mixed with a turbulent nausea. When the seatbelt sign dinged on, I remembered hearing some-one talk about an airline pilot he knew: the pilot said flights were hours of absolute boredom broken up by moments of sheer terror. I put my face between my knees to steady my stomach and pictured the vertical kilometres that stretched from my shoes to the ocean.

When my uncle Roberto, Nonno, and I arrived in Italy, Nonno had decided it was best that we adjust to the time difference right away and stay up until it was nighttime in Rome. Nonno, anxious about being only a day away from his childhood home, the Ferrari farm, and about seeing some of his relatives again, said that he wasn't tired and told me that he was too excited to eat. He hadn't planned on coming on this trip, his third and final one, until just a week before we were set to leave. His first trip, in the mid-1970s, more than twenty years after he had emigrated, was with his brother-in-law. This time, Nanni Rose told him to go with us, to show me around their hometowns and to speak Calabrese when my uncle's Italian wouldn't do. She herself would stay at home. She stuck to the vow she had made the day she stepped off the *Andrea Doria*: she would never return.

Nonno and Uncle had made this same trip once together some years before, a father-son bonding that adhered to the order of things. They never searched for Rosina among Nonno's old haunts, but this time, the three generations together would look for whatever it was that I wanted to find, Nonno said. I felt privileged to step into the Old Country as the first female from Nanni Rose's branch of our family. I was returning for Nanni Rose, and I would be beside her husband, my Nonno Filippo, when he said goodbye to his hometown for the final time.

I hadn't noticed the sun when I sank into bed, exhausted from the day of travel and full day in Rome without sleep. I felt my chest move up and down; I was breathing as if asleep, but I couldn't stop thinking about the sun pinned to the night sky. Reality bordered dream, and I was in some limbo space between Edmonton and the Old Country, and between a world I'd imagined and one that I was about to enter. Those skies I'd fixed with false clouds and constructed sunsets would soon spread out before me.

In the morning, as we stepped out of the hotel on our way back to the airport to take the short flight to Calabria, I saw a large orange circular sign, not as bright in the daylight, that signalled airport parking. I decided not to tell anyone why I was so tired.

No trains go directly into the villages of Maione, Altilia, or Grimaldi in Calabria, so we decided to fly into Salerno and rent a car to take us there. While we waited on the tarmac in the stifling plane, we heard that ten other planes stood ahead of us. Still so many miles between me and that world I'd imagined, that site of all the *c'era una voltas*, the once-upon-a-times, of the family stories.

After moving ahead plane-length by plane-length, we finally pulled forward and tugged into the air. My stomach rose and fell until the plane steadied out. We were so far above the quilted fields and snaking rivers that I could not distinguish land from water or sky. I felt like I was making a counter-journey, a movement back to the place that so many left for Canada. As we approached Salerno, I saw the coastline and thought of young Rose with her brother Vittorio on the *Andrea Doria*. The ship would push away from Italy until they were so far away they weren't sure if they could still see it on the horizon.

I glanced over at Nonno, who was bending to see through the small window. Dressed in his white T-shirt with Canada written across the chest, he squirmed left and right to see past the wing. He looked over at me and patted his shirt flat. "I'm so glad I packed this shirt. I also packed a jar of instant coffee, the kind you get at Superstore."

"I think instant coffee tastes gross. I only drink it when I go camping." I laughed.

"Ah, that espresso stuff they drink here. *That* is bad. But *they* just love it. It is all about what you get used to," Nonno said while shaking his head. "But instant coffee is the best." He dropped his wicker sun hat onto his head and folded his hands on his lap.

"How's your stomach feeling?"

"Not great, but I'll make it," I said. I reclined my seat and stared straight ahead.

"Do you need water? Want to switch seats? Your Nanni, she gets sick on planes and in cars just like you, so I know what it's like. She doesn't like to travel anymore. And I'll let you know a little secret."

"What's the secret?"

"Your nanni said I had to look after you, and if I don't . . ." He trailed off while making a swiping motion across his neck with his thumb. "Dead meat."

He peeked out the window again. "Almost there now," Nonno exhaled.

I imagined him fifty-six years earlier. With a suitcase in hand and an unstamped passport, he inches closer to Canada, to the grid of streets and avenues in an unknown city, while he sails away from Calabria, a village whose hills he could navigate in the dark.

It was a quiet ride to Altilia as we each took in the landscape: small hillside villages, narrow roadways, rolling vista after rolling vista. We each had different connections to the Old Country and different reasons to visit. I tried to imagine what it was like for Nonno to see a place again after so long way but still know its intricacies: the places to get water, to find shade, to hide, to pray. Almost immediately, the Calabrese fell from his mouth like liquid and reminded me that this was his first world. When I considered that at age seventy-three, he'd spent more of his life in Canada than Calabria, his ability to find this language again spoke of that learned connection between signifier and signified: words and referents. *Mamma* and Carmela Ferrari. *Villaggio* and Altilia. *Amore* and Rose Russo. This was the place at the base of all memory, the place everything else came from.

Uncle served as the bridge between generations. The one who could translate because he'd learned and could recall at least some of the Italian he had known as a child. He would raise his hand against a conversation, to pause it, and share the important parts with me. He was there to keep his promise to his mother, my Nanni Rose, to make sure Nonno ate vegetables and slowed down because he was his *dottore* and so he had no choice. And Uncle, like me, was an outsider, and could help interpret the world that belonged to our ancestors against the place where we were born. As my godfather, Uncle mentioned more than once that he would never have missed coming *here* with me, doing *this* with me.

We twisted and turned up the narrow road to Altilia. Each bend was a complete fishhook, until we arrived at the top. Uncle put the car in park along G. Marsico Street. When we opened our doors, the heat tumbled over us, thick and heavy. We entered Calabria during the afternoon siesta, and the village was as silent as if we were visiting a forgotten historic site. Since no one else was around, I could brush my hands along crumbling concrete walls, teeter on the uneven cobblestone road, and examine the perfect shadow of a curly lamppost against a brick wall. Uncle Roberto nodded when I said, "I can't believe we are here. This place does not seem real."

"I know. I felt the same way. Come look out at the edge of the hill."

Nonno leaned against the metal railing.

"Over there," Nonno pointed. "See, near where there is now a curvy road? That small white square? That's my house."

I squinted into what looked like a hazy, stretched-out oil painting thick with olive, pine, and emerald brushstrokes. Calabria.

A thin squiggle of clouds poked out from the line of hills that separated the greens from the sky. I traced the line that Nonno had drawn in the air between the highway and a hill and I saw it: his childhood home. *I'm here?*

"We'll have to go down there sometime this week. I'll show you."

"I'd love to see it. And the house where Rosina lived for all those years. On the hill?" I imagined that this story-place was just beyond a hill—just out of view—as I leaned against the railing and stared at the edges of this expanse.

"Every house is on a hill," Nonno said. "But I know the one. Maybe you can see it from up here."

We all walked across the road and leaned over a stone wall where we had a view of Maione. The village formed a near oval. It contained houses that, from a few kilometres away, looked nearly identical. White houses with orange roofs. An image you'd find in a calendar. A road bordered the town, hemmed it in, but all around dense fields of thick, green trees grew up and down hills. Fields as rolling as the waves of the Atlantic.

"Rosina lived just outside of the village of Maione, just like I lived just outside of Altilia. We lived on farms. I don't think you can see their place from this spot, but we'll find it." Nonno put his hands flat on the top of the wall and lifted himself to get a better view.

"Yeah, we will get to the house, even if we have to do some serious investigating," Uncle assured me. I stared down at the clusters of trees and the overgrown pathways. "But make no mistake, we will see snakes." He frowned.

Only a valley, a dip in the earth, separated the two villages. There was only a valley between young Filippo Ferrari and Rose Russo. Between Nonno's family, who owned their own land, and Nanni Rose's, who worked other people's land. Between abundance and hunger. And now, half a century later, between Maione and me.

"Let's go. I told Tonino we'd arrive in the early afternoon," Nonno said. When I turned around, he was almost back to the car.

"Back down the fishhook roads," Uncle said and swerved his hand through the air.

"So," I asked, while visualizing the inky lines that I'd drawn connecting one person to another. "Tonino's mother was Adelina Russo? One of Rosina's four daughters?" I imagined a line downwards from Rosina to Adelina and another from Adelina downwards to Tonino.

"Yes, Adelina."

"And she died just one year after Rosina. In 1970?"

"Yes, I think so."

After I had found those funeral cards and gathered more information, I'd discovered that Rosina's other three daughters had died before her: Terracina in 1966, Maria in 1967, and Palmira, the one without a card, sometime before 1969. On the family tree, I had circled Rosina's losses in red. First, her husband, Giovanni. Then everyone she lived with in the farmhouse before emigration: Generoso, her baby boy, Michelina, his wife, and their children, her grandchildren: Giovanni, Rose, Vittorio, Maria, and Maurizio. I imagined the house folding in on itself. The fields swallowing it whole. And then her three daughters. I considered writing the dates of her losses next to the circles, but that didn't seem to matter.

We turned into a curve partway down the hill to Francesca and Tonino's house. We pulled the car up to the bottom of a long, gated driveway, but we didn't have to ring the buzzer. Through the gate, I saw the largest and one of the newest-looking houses I'd seen in Altilia. The gate slid open, and we drove up to a three-storey, tan, and rust-tiled house. I'd heard that the three brothers remaining in Calabria had inherited much of the land, but I had not expected such a large house in such a small village.

I climbed the steps up the side of the house where Francesca stood with one hand on her square hip and the other outstretched. She was dressed in a bright red tank top and grey sweat shorts, and her short dyed brown hair, a square cut, sprouted grey roots. Her booming voice filled the yard, "Ah! Buongiorno! Mario! Eh!" she said to my grandfather as they hugged.

I'd never heard him called Mario before, and it was jolting, especially in Francesca's heavy voice. But then, I remembered the story about his father writing Filippo Mario on his birth certificate, even though his superstitious mother had wanted him to be called

Mario to thwart an early death. I guess the false first name, the only name he had known until his first day of school, had stuck. I looked at him, small in Francesca's embrace: Nonno Mario. It seemed fitting that in his first language, he had a different first name. I attached signifier to signified within the framework of this world new to me: from Nonno Filippo to Mario Ferrari. From old Italian grandfather with a grey moustache who lives just off Yellowhead Trail to young tailor with dark hair skipping across a river to talk to Rose.

Tonino emerged through the brown plastic beads hanging in the doorway between the covered porch and kitchen and pulled me in, his bony frame hard against my own. He was shorter than Francesca and soft-spoken. The longer that I looked at him, nearly eye to eye since we were almost the same height, the more I saw myself: boney knees and ankles, hard pointy elbows, oval face and glasses.

"Buongiorno! Buongiorno!" he said while nodding his head and smiling so wide that I already felt comfortable, even if I would have to do charades.

Francesca was already in the kitchen pulling out glasses and bottles of water and cola. We sat down for a drink. The shutters over the kitchen's patio doors cast long-lined shadows across the blue-checkered table and everyone seated around it.

Uncle explained to Tonino that I had found the picture of

Rosina, and that I wanted to know more about her, see where she lived and find her gravesite.

Tonino leaned toward me, tapped the top of my hand, and smiled.

Tonino and Francesca showed us our rooms in the walkout basement, while Francesca explained—and Uncle translated—that they had lived in Rome for twenty-one years, but they had to move; she had too many allergies in the city. She rattled off her list of self-diagnosed allergies and explained that when she felt tight in the chest, she'd just signal to Tonino and he'd drive her to the ocean, where she could breathe again.

Francesca was born in Rome and most of her family still lived in the north. Tonino had gone there for work when he was young, and that's where they met. Francesca starts to tell the story but does not slow down for Uncle to translate it for me. He keeps turning his head from Francesca back to me while he tries to relay what she is saying. She was carrying a bag of groceries down a long set of stairs. Somewhere in Rome. Tonino was walking in the opposite direction. Somehow, he was not looking or something and he smacked into her. Spilled her groceries everywhere. There's food all over. Their eyes met. She looked down at him, and she said, "What the hell? Am I so damn ugly that you didn't notice me?" Tonino said, "Yes! You are! Watch where you are walking!" They were never apart after that. They moved south, back to Tonino's hometown. They built this house on the land Tonino's father, Saverio, had owned. They wanted a big house so they could welcome any guests who visited. Saverio worked in Canada. Miette Hot Springs in Alberta.

I watched as Francesca motioned her arm through the air, signalling just how long her father-in-law had been in Alberta.

Mom had told me about camping trips to see her uncle Saverio, who was living in a train car while working on the railroads. She remembered him buying all the children ice cream, any size they wanted. After twenty-three years, Saverio returned to Calabria with the money he had saved and purchased more of the land that surrounded what he had owned before he left. Today, what Saverio acquired is divided among his three sons: Tonino, Dario, and Amadeo. Their land sprawls across most of Altilia.

Uncle turned to Nonno, and in English asked, "Did Saverio ever have a girlfriend in Miette?"

"Oh. Yes, of course. He was there for twenty-three years. He sent money home for his family."

I raised my eyebrows, but Uncle just shrugged.

"Ah, what do you expect? That's a long time!" Nonno said.

When Tonino and Francesca went back upstairs, we zipped open our suitcases to search for fresh clothes. I threw bottled water and sunscreen into a backpack. Uncle stood in the doorway of his room and continued translating what I'd missed. "Francesca also said that when she moved here the other women from the village gossiped about her wearing shorts. People were more liberal in the North and in the big cities like Rome."

"So, she just continued to wear them?" I asked while reconsidering the shorts and tank top I was wearing.

"Yep. She also explained that she does not care to wear a bra, especially at home, and she really didn't care what they had to say about that."

"Good for her!"

"She also swears, dirty, dirty words, when she's telling any story."

"Some things are universal. I caught those!" I laughed.

Tonino pulled the car out of the garage to the sliding door of the basement. I rubbed sunscreen on my shoulders and face as the thirty-five-degree heat soaked into my skin, then slid into the back seat.

Tonino was driving us to the cemetery in Grimaldi to find Rosina's gravesite. I wasn't certain if she was buried in Maione, Altilia, or Grimaldi, but I'd always imagined it was in Maione since she had lived there for so many years and since she was the only one to remain. I'd imagined her gravestone with the family name would stand in for those relatives who would be buried in sprawling city cemeteries. It was easy to imagine that she was buried in Maione because that's the last place I can see her: standing in the doorway of the empty farmhouse.

Nanni Rose had never returned and never saw Rosina's gravesite. She said that she wasn't even sure there was a grave to return to.

Tonino explained that he knew Rosina was buried in Grimaldi because soon after Generoso and Michelina and all of their children emigrated, Rosina had also had to leave the farmhouse in Maione. She moved in with her daughter Palmira's daughter—Sisina. Sisina lived in the town of Grimaldi, just a few kilometres north.

"Will I be able to talk with Sisina?" I asked, desperate to know what the rest of Rosina's life had been like and grateful for a living link.

"Ah. I don't know. Sisina's an old woman now, Jessica," Nonno explained from the front seat.

I leaned forward between the front seats. "Could we visit her? See if she would be up for talking?"

"Sometimes when people grow old, they don't remember much. I think it would be pointless now."

I turned to Uncle.

"We'll go see," Uncle stepped in. "Just see how she is. If she's up for talking, we'll talk. If she's not, we will just say hello."

"Ah, I think it's pointless!" Nonno threw his hands up and let them fall to his lap.

Tonino stopped near a tall, thin metal crucifix and jumped out. I wasn't sure if I was ready to see Rosina's gravestone, but at the same time, I wanted something tangible. Something that wasn't a story that ebbed and flowed according to whose memory she was contained within. Something that wasn't a document, that left no room for footnotes, endnotes, side stories. There is something real about kneeling before someone's resting spot, about the stone jutting up through the earth to mark their place. This is as close as I could come to visiting Rosina, my great-great-grandmother. I thought of that time, years ago now, when I sat in my sister's kitchen asking questions about Rosina. Those second-hand stories Melissa had heard through Nanni Rose seemed so removed from me now.

Wide slabs of cement led down from the cemetery's wrought-iron gate at the top of the hill. On either side of this staircase were marble tombs, rows that stretched out to either side of the cemetery stacked four-plots high, with the older gravesites along the bottom and the newer ones built on top. Each individual plot was marked with its own metal plaque and black-and-white photo. Altogether, they formed long houses that contain residents with various surnames, all beneath one marble roof and between two marble walls on either side. Some of the older graves displayed post-mortem photos, likely because a picture had not been taken during the individual's life, though, with open eyes staged to look lifelike.

We didn't find her there. We left after reading name after name and looking at picture after picture. Tonino shook his head and shrugged as we all got back into the car and made our way to Aquino's house in Maione. Everyone chatted in Italian. In my mind, I kept repeating, *Rosina, Rosina, Rosina*, in rhythm with the hum of the car and the rise and fall of words that I couldn't make out.

Aquino's house was at the top of a long set of cement stairs that was most easily reached by driving the wrong way down a one-way street. Red peppers had been strung to the railing to dry and bunches of purple grapes hung over the front porch, creating privacy and shade. Aquino's wife, Giuseppina, emerged through the beaded doorway first and hugged Nonno, then Uncle and me. She had glasses and drinks on the porch table and was pulling chairs around it before Nonno had finished introducing me to Aquino. I made another connection in my mind, another inky line down from Rosina to her daughter Maria, and from Maria to Maria's son Aquino.

While everyone chatted, the only familiar words I could hear were *Cah-nada* and *Nah-na Ro-seena*. Each time, after they spoke of Rosina, they'd all look at me and smile.

"What are you talking about?" I whispered to Uncle.

"Oh, just telling them about your curiosity about Rosina. How you found that picture and want to know more about her."

I looked over at Aquino, whose dark skin and coarse black hair made him look much younger than he was. He had to be in his sixties, but his wrinkles were hidden behind his grey stubble.

Aquino turned to me and told me a few words he had learned when he worked in Canada. After listening to him speak Italian, the words that came out of his mouth, in almost unaccented English, transformed him for a moment into someone else.

"Chair. Table. Tree." Aquino laughed and took another sip of his beer.

"Birra," I said and pointed to Aquino's drink.

"Ah! Sì!"

We went inside before we left. The floor was white marble and felt cool on my feet. There was a coat rack in the corner, and above it, a plaque that said Canada, with a postcard of Edmonton and a tiny plastic Canadian flag. I looked at all the photos hanging on their walls, and pointed to one that I recognized from the funeral cards I went through at Nanni and Nonno's place—the younger-looking woman with dark hair who looked off to the side.

"Maria?" I asked Aquino.

"Sì, mia mamma," he replied.

He pointed to the man beside her. "Mio papà."

Those papers, stuffed in the plastic bag, were suddenly infused with meaning. Here was Aquino. And Maria no longer a distant relative in another place, no longer so far from me, she was his *mamma* and I was here in *Maione*.

On the way home, Uncle explained that Aquino was going to take us back to the cemetery in Grimaldi because he was certain that Rosina was there.

Her photo, in an oval metal frame, is fastened to a piece of smooth marble. The marble is secured between two rows of rust-coloured bricks secured by bulging lines of cement; the narrow plot could only fit bones or ashes. I wonder if she was first buried in the ground in the centre of the cemetery, her body lowered into the earth that she spent her lifetime working. This square of soil is so dry that only a few blades of brown grass poke up around the perimeter. The roots of a huge oak tree gnaw up through the packed ground—yellowed, curled bones.

Families with more money stay together in private tombs with doors that lock. Surnames run like welcome signs across the door. Surnames of people who owned the land they farmed. Wide pots are filled with real flowers that bend under the heat. Tiny red hydrangea petals are scattered across the doorsteps. From the top of the cemetery, these tombs, with peaked roofs covered in orange terracotta tiles, follow the curve of the hill—house next to house.

Attached to the side of one of the marble communal rows is a small covered area where Rosina's gravesite sits below two cleared-out plots. These rectangular spaces are empty except for a few stray flowers and clumps of brick and cement. I place my hand on the cool cement bottom of an empty plot to steady myself as I bend down to get closer to her gravesite.

I yank my hand out when I realize that before the space was cleared out, a stranger could have been resting there for years, and ashes could have sunk into the cracks of the cement to be left undisturbed, sheltered beneath a marble roof, in the tiny corner of the graveyard. I crouch down, and there she is—Rosina, in a narrow hallway of souls in Grimaldi, Calabria.

Aquino walks over to where I am crouching and points up to a stone tucked in the corner of the wall across from Rosina.

I stand up next to him and look up.

"Mia mamma."

"Sì. Maria," I say softly.

Aquino nods his head slowly and steps back out into the bright sun.

Here in the shade beneath the marble roof, shadowed by the fake flowers, is a picture of Rosina I have never seen.

She is older and smaller than she was in the photo with her arm on the chair, almost smiling. But here, I'm not sure that she is alive. Her eyes are darker, sunken. The photo, covered by a thick piece of glass, makes it difficult to see Rosina. I can tell that she is wearing a different black dress or shirt with a thin pressed collar and her hair, pulled back or short, is more white than in the first photo.

As I read the stone, loss tightens my throat and makes my heart pound. A deep beat. I've never felt as close to Nanni Rose as I do here in Calabria. Here, her loss, that final goodbye in 1955, rushes over me.

BENINCASA ROSINA.
Aprile 2, 1883–Luglio 28, 1969

DODICI

borderlines the separations between one place and another

I walk up the cemetery's steps to the top of the hill, where Nonno leans against the car and talks to Aquino. With pointed fingers, they draw maps in the air and repeat *no* and *sì* over and over.

"Okay! Andiamo. Andiamo," Nonno says as he swings open my door.

"Grazie, Nonno."

He slides into the passenger seat of Aquino's tiny blue car parked just ahead. I am certain the old car does not have air conditioning like our rental and yell, "Drink some of your water," just as he slams his door shut.

Uncle blasts the air, and we flick and turn dials until the cool air reaches us. We coast downhill toward Maione, following Aquino to his house so that he can tell Giuseppina that he will be away for the afternoon. Their air-maps will lead us to the Maione farmhouse.

Aquino strides up a few of the cement stairs leading to his place, but then, while standing on his toes, stops and yells into the window where his wife emerges. With one hand on the window frame, she leans her body forward; the other hand holds a checkered dishtowel that she shakes at him as he talks. Her white hair is bright in the afternoon light and she smiles and waves down at us. She nods, then the window is empty, and he rushes back to the car.

"So, why is it going to be so hard to find?" I ask Uncle as we jerk and twist through the streets to keep up with the old car.

"It's not so much hard to find as hard to get to. Everything around here was abandoned. Now it's overgrown. No one has any reason to go to these empty farmhouses. Oh, and there are snakes. Slithery, slimy, sneaky snakes."

The day before, we had stopped at Amadeo's place—Tonino's little brother. Amadeo, well over six-feet tall, towered over Tonino as they greeted each other with a backslapping hug. After hugging Nonno, Amadeo placed his hand on my shoulder, and Nonno introduced me by spreading out his five fingers to list his five children in order, before pointing back at his thumb, my mother, and then over to me.

When Amadeo realized we were still standing in the front doorway, he gestured toward the living room, rolling his hand and calling us in.

The living room was bright with sponged peach walls and a gold-coloured rope-like crown moulding. A big flat-screen TV sat on a brick shelf in one corner of the room, and beside it, a gas fireplace, and a shelf that contained knickknacks like a saint in a brown robe and a shiny white vase. There was a gold-framed oil painting of flowers on one wall, and landscape prints hung above the dining table. The grey marble floor felt cool on my feet as I walked across the room to take a glass of juice that Amadeo's wife, Maria, had set out for us.

Uncle started to translate snippets of conversations from around the living room. I'd learned that Amadeo's two children, both in their early thirties, had difficulty finding work. Amadeo's daughter, Emilia, had attended university in Rome and then spent eight years trying to get a job with her PHD in psychology. She eventually found a position in Cosenza, the nearest city to her hometown. It was too far to commute between the city and Altilia, so she had to move. Amadeo's son, Saverio, named after his grandfather who had spent so many years working in Miette, was unemployed and lived at home. Since Saverio was only a few years older than me, I wished I could sit and chat with him: ask him what it was like to grow up in Altilia, what stories he had heard about his relatives in Alberta. We were a part of the same generation of Rosina's descendants, and we knew nothing of each other. All we could do was smile, nod, and pass a plate of eggplant and pitcher of juice.

From Amadeo's top balcony, I had looked down through white clotheslines decorated with coloured pegs; I looked across the countryside, where one farm blended into another. The walls of empty houses poked up through treetops and suggested that there had been individual sections of land but that the border between farms had blurred over time as roots curled into roots. It was as if— once abandoned—all the land had pulled together. Consequently, distinctions between areas had blurred for those emigrants who made their way to Edmonton and other Canadian cities. They formed groups of Italian Canadians despite cultural and linguistic differences, and despite having identified with their village before identifying with the Italian nation. They pulled together.

I sat on a leather couch listening to the voices around the room and then Uncle, after chatting with Saverio, came and joined me. Uncle explained to Amadeo that we were going to find the house because I was curious about Rosina's life: about who she was and where she had lived. Amadeo looked over at me and nodded before he left the room. He came back with something in his hand. He leaned toward me and handed me a five-by-seven photo on a thick paper that looked pocket-sized in his huge hands. The glossy image, with rich blacks and shiny greys, was Rosina—that hand on her hip, the other resting on the back of that wooden chair. Another copy, kept in another glass cabinet: this time along with an *Inglese–Italiano Dizionario* and books about the history of Calabria. He asked Uncle if I could send him a copy of the family tree, once I had filled out all the lines. I agreed, and Amadeo pinched my cheek and held his palm against my face.

On our way to find the house, we drive down a narrow, unpaved road surrounded by gnarled olive trees. Uncle explains that olive trees must be maintained with regular pruning or they will not produce any fruit. Many of these olive trees are barren even though it's almost September. As we continue, tall dry grasses poke out and press flat against our windows. We thump over roots and holes as we lurch along the narrowing road. The dirt gives way to thick packed grass and we are no longer on a road at all.

Branches shriek and snap against the car doors, but Aquino keeps on going. His tiny old car bumps along the rutted ground. I wonder if he and Nonno are reminiscing about walking down these pathways as two young boys carrying baskets of olives to be crushed, or about who lived where and for how long. The two older men seem oblivious to the squeaks of the car as they continue forward; they are talking with their hands, wide, sweeping gestures that we watch though their back window. Uncle brakes when a cluster of twigs slaps against our windshield, leaving dry leaves in the wipers. We wave to them to stop, and honk our horn until their brake lights flash through the overgrowth.

"This is not driveable!" Uncle shouts as he leans out the driver's door.

Aquino seems to agree: he and Nonno climb out. We walk ahead on what I can tell was once a pathway. There are banks on either side with even taller grasses and nettles. Aquino points down the hill.

"This was where his parents lived. This is his mother, Maria's, house. This isn't far from where Rosina lived," Nonno explains while clomping toward it.

I look over at Aquino, a rather thick, tough-looking man with sun-browned skin and hands on his hips, and think of the moment we shared in that tiny hallway at the cemetery. With his hand by his side, he had pointed a finger upwards, flashed his eyes up at his mama's grave, and then looked at me.

"So, the family stayed close together, even after the daughters got married? Maria stayed near her mom?"

"Oh. Of course. Well, until emigration."

Months earlier, I had met Aquino's younger brother Pino, who lived in Edmonton. He'd described this area to me, explained that houses were usually small and open inside. The building, now only four fieldstone walls buried in wheat, was once a popular place. Other village residents from Maione and Altilia came here to use the grinding mill. Maria and her husband, Antonio, Aquino's mother and father, received food in exchange for the use of their machine: sacks of flour, jars of olive oil, fresh figs.

I smile at Aquino, wishing I could say something more to him about his childhood home and about my meeting with his brother Pino in Edmonton. The day before, when Uncle asked Aquino if he could tell me any stories about Rosina, he seemed shy, shrugged his shoulders and avoided eye contact. He just said something like, "I don't know what to say. She was a kind and strong woman." He was probably more comfortable with my forced silence.

I nod as Nonno explains the process of exchanging goods to me in English. I watch Aquino wade through the wheat. The thick stalks snap under his heavy feet as he moves.

"You know, Jessica, I'm sure it's hard to imagine, but this whole area used to be cultivated. Perfect rows of plants. Grapevines down the hills—line after line. It was like one big garden," Nonno said, swiping his arm through the air as if to clear-cut.

The trees reach into one another behind the house and create a leafy wall. Some of the branches lean against the roofless house. I find it easier to imagine that the trees, wheat, and grasses will eventually swallow the house whole than to envision the area cultivated.

We get back into the cars and turn around. The Maione farmhouse is not far up the path in the opposite direction.

When Uncle and I are inside the car, I ask, "Why did we come this way?"

"I guess Aquino wanted to show you where his mom had lived."

We turn around and drive along a cliff. The road seems wide enough for our car, but it curls up a hill so it is difficult to see what's ahead. I half expect that around the bend will be Rosina's house as I've imagined it: a small house on the hill, a field of yellow wheat trimmed at the edges, and the river, a border between their land and the rest, with firmly placed footholds to cross.

Our tires scrape against the rocks that jut out of the side of the road, jolting me from my daydream. In another instant, bare branches stretch across the windshield.

"Oh my god!" I yell as the branches shriek up and over the roof when we drive through them. I picture the tiny white lines scraped into the paintwork of the black car.

I look out my window and down the cliff. The brush might cushion our fall, but it is a long way down.

"Should we look at the damage?" I ask.

"There is nowhere to turn around! What's the point?"

We all get out, and Aquino points ahead, where a stone wall juts between thick bushes. He shrugs. I wonder how we'll ever get the cars back down the cliff. I worry about the bill we'll receive from the rental company as I smudge my thumb along the lines in the black paint. They won't rub off. But I want to see what's past the wall. The house has to be somewhere up ahead.

"Come, Jessica!" Nonno says and continues up the hill to the wall. "It's right over there! I don't know why there is a wall here."

As I step out, a thin black snake rustles under the brush and over the clumps of dirt on the edge of the cliff.

"I just saw a snake!" I shriek.

"I. Told. You," Uncle answers and leans back against the car to scan the ground.

Nonno and Aquino are already at the wall, so I plunge forward. There it is: a rectangular stone house in the distance. Only the top of a sidewall and a small area of the front are visible. Past the wall a barbed-wire fence—rows of silver wire—stretches up and over a hill.

"Where is the river?"

"Down there." Nonno points down the hill in front of the house. "But it's almost bone-dry because of the time of year and because no one is watering this land. Nothing is going back into it."

"I imagined it right close to the house."

"Why?"

"I'm not sure."

All of the stories seem distorted as I reimagine them here. Twist them to fit. A palimpsest: the river as I imagined, gushing with years of reflections, overlaid on a dry track that tapers into trees.

"Is that river the place where you crossed with those eggs in your pockets?"

"Yes. Right down there, and I was wearing my suit too! But it was a different place then, there's no way to get there."

The house, made of fieldstone and mortar, seems to jut out of the ground. The thatched roof has decayed. I wish I could get closer, but I am sure that anything inside has long ago become dust.

It was dark by the time we headed back to Tonino and Francesca's house. As we curled up the hill, our headlights—long yellow beams broken by the curve of the road—were the only source of light. Nonno rode in the back seat, insisting that I sit in the front so that the twisty roads wouldn't make me sick. He started snoring within a few minutes. A small cement wall was built along the cliffside, and I followed the bend as the car moved slowly alongside it until Uncle slammed on the brakes and we all heaved forward.

A dog, with long golden hair, sat in the centre of the road between the two beams.

"That was close," Uncle said while gripping the wheel and leaning forward to get a better look at the dog.

"Stray dogs. Nowhere to go but the middle of the road," Nonno added as he cleared his throat.

Eventually, the dog got up and sauntered to the side. I watched him until he was no bigger than a pinhead in the side mirror. I was tired when we arrived back at Tonino and Francesca's, but Amadeo and his wife, Maria, had come over. An empty bottle of red wine sat on the table and another had just been uncorked. It appeared as though they had just finished dinner. Francesca's pink rubber gloves lay on the side of the sink, and a basket of hard bread remained on the counter.

We all sat around the table, except for Francesca, who was in the living room yelling at the soccer game.

Soon everyone started discussing soccer politics, except for Nonno, who just laughed and leaned across the table to tell me that clearly, they had it all wrong, because the only sport worth arguing about was hockey. Talk became so heated that people lifted off their seats and then sat back down, red-faced.

"Are they actually mad at each other?" I asked Uncle, who was just finishing one glass of wine and pouring another.

"Oh, no! They're just loud. Wait until Tonino brings up the Fascists."

When Tonino noticed that the bottle of wine was empty, he jumped up and started counting how many shot glasses he would need. He put tiny Niagara Falls glasses on the table. Nonno picked one up and bounced it in his palm. "These are from their trip to Canada. I think in '95."

Francesca lifted a huge bottle of homemade unlabelled liquid from the china cabinet. The bright yellow limoncello sloshed around in the bottle as she ambled across the living room to the kitchen. She filled the glasses and set them down in front of us. Everyone held them up and said, "Chin, chin!" before drinking. The limoncello burned all the way to the bottom of my stomach, a long line from my throat to my belly.

"Why do we say *chin chin* and not *ching ching*? Aren't we trying to mimic the sound of glasses?" I whisper to Uncle.

"In Calabrese they don't have the *-ing* sound."

Francesca explained in her thick Calabrese that she'd tried to make some limoncello when they visited Canada, but it was impossible to find one hundred proof alcohol. Uncle shook his head, then said to Nonno, "When Francesca talks fast, I can't make out her Calabrese."

"You can't learn Calabrese in university." Nonno laughed. "But your Italian will help us in Rome where I sometimes don't understand a damn thing."

"Oh, Mario! You'd be just fine," I joked and chinged my glass against his.

"Hey! That's Nonno Mario to you! And when we are back home, it's Nonno Filippo!"

Before long, the Italian and Calabrese, against the clinking and cheers for the soccer game, swirled together. I couldn't make out anything. Tonino held the large bottle in his hands and gestured to me by holding it up and tilting it.

"No, grazie! Sto bene," I said while I rubbed my belly.

I pulled out my Hilroy notebook from my purse at my feet and opened it to the family tree that I'd been building. I had Uncle help me ask Tonino and Amadeo to fill in some dates. They went through the list of Rosina and Giovanni's children: Terracina, Adelina, Maria, Palmira, and Generoso. After ending at Generoso, they pointed at us, his descendants. But then, in a hushed voice, they started talking about something else and, after a while, I gathered some*one* else.

"What's going on?" I asked Uncle.

He held up his finger and leaned closer to the other side of the table to try to listen. "I don't know. I can't follow."

The TV was flashing in the corner of the room as the screen changed between different news stories.

"Dad," Uncle said, while tapping Nonno on the arm. "Are they talking about another child? Another baby . . . of Rosina's?"

I listened for familiar words, but they all ran together.

Nonno answered Uncle in Calabrese, and I tapped my hand against the table and asked again.

"In English, please!" I pleaded to Nonno over the revived soccer discussion.

"Yes. Apparently, she had another baby boy. Generoso wasn't her only son."

"But Generoso was the youngest child and only boy. That's

why Rosina eventually moved in with him. He became the man of the house . . ."

"This baby boy died when he was seventeen days old. He was born sometime before Generoso."

I felt the limoncello sink down and my eyes fill with tears. I stared at the wineglass beside me, half a sip left. I twirled the stem between my thumb and forefinger; the booming voices from around the table spun into one solid sound.

"What was his name?" I imagined Rosina holding her first baby boy, rocking him at home, in that place behind the wall and barbed-wire lines. In that place buried in trees and beneath years of decay. In that house that belonged to her and Giovanni, before his heart gave out, and he was gone. They didn't have a doctor nearby, or a clinic or hospital, so I imagine the baby was at home on that seventeenth day. Rosina didn't give birth five times, just like Nanni Rose and Mom. She gave birth six times.

Nonno didn't answer. Uncle asked him the same question in Italian.

"Emilio Antonio," he answered to Uncle.

"Did Nanni know about this?" I asked Uncle, who just shook his head no.

I imagined another inky red circle on the family tree. This time, around seventeen-day-old Emilio Antonio.

T R E D I C I

zenith the point in the sky directly above the
observer

I unfolded the photocopied sheet of the *Situazione di Famiglia del Sig. Russo Generoso fu Giovanni* and pointed to Rosina's name across line eight.

"Ah, Sì. Benincasa," said the blond woman. She flipped through the folios of village records, running her finger across the large yellowed pages. She had been confused about what we were searching for until I pulled out that paper, a photocopy of the one Nanni had saved the day they cleaned out her parents' house.

Someone in The Scattered had told me that in order to get records from any town hall it was necessary to bring a resident of the village because the records were not distributed very easily; they explained that the workers only offered typed-up versions, not photocopies of the originals. Tonino agreed to accompany us. The Comune di Altilia, a yellow stucco building at the top of the village, held the records for both Altilia and Maione. Spines of green and black canvas folios were visible through a stone archway just behind the woman's desk.

"Shouldn't everything be entered into a computer?" I whispered to Uncle and nudged him to look at the collection of folios.

"To top it off, it seems you have to search by date of the event—birth, marriage, death—to locate the right folio, and then you have to search through them," he said while glancing through the archway.

"So . . . if you don't know the date before you start searching . . . ?"

"You don't get the records."

"No. No," the woman said and shut the last folio she had pulled off the shelves. I envisioned the long cursive letters inside, pressed against one another.

Tonino shook his head at me, and Nonno explained that there were no records on Rosina Benincasa here.

"Nothing?"

"No records."

Nonno, still unsure about visiting Rosina's niece Sisina, agreed that we should at least go and check the Comune di Grimaldi for records. He suggested that after checking there for records we go spend the day on the beach in Amantea. He repeated that Sisina wouldn't know anything. That she forgets things. That talking to her would be pointless. A waste of a chance to dip our feet in the ocean.

As we were equipped with my photocopied list of the people who lived in the house with Rosina—our passport—Tonino decided to go home for lunch with Francesca. We turned the wrong way down the one-way street and parked the car at Aquino's and then walked up through winding side streets, crevices we moved through in single file.

We reached the Comune, a large, unpainted cement building, in the corner of a square of villas and a worn brick church with a heavy wooden door. In the middle of the square stretched a star made of cubes of white marble placed in the cobblestones.

We waited as the clerk flipped through the pages. I noticed a manila envelope stamped and addressed to someone in Vancouver, British Columbia, on her desk. I wondered if inside there were someone's family records, certificates of marriage or death. Documents lost through migration. Eventually, she shook her head of big brown curls, pulled her glasses off, and looked at us. "Niente."

"Nothing," I repeated.

Just as she was about to pull the book off her desk, she stopped and flattened her hand against one page. I stared at the pages but couldn't make out the cursive Italian. She said something to Nonno, and then he turned to me. "Okay. They don't have a Rosina Benincasa. They do have a birth record of a Rosina *Vienincasa* born in 1883."

"*Vienincasa?* Same year . . . Is it? Well, that must be her."

Her name, sounds that had signified matriarch, midwife, non-migrant, and mother, became momentarily detached. Rosina Vienincasa: a new set of syllables to practise. Rosina *Vienin*casa. I looked at Nonno Filippo, now Nonno Mario in Calabria, as he asked the woman to look up Rosina Vienincasa's death certificate. It was still her. I tried to reshape the trajectory of Rosina's life. I placed my finger on the top of the wooden desk and drew a G, M, G. If she had lived with Sisina at the end of her life, and there was a record here of her birth in Grimaldi, she was born in Grimaldi and died in Grimaldi, although she spent most of her life in Maione on the farm: a lifetime on the land only stories could testify to.

Why didn't her gravestone match these records? How fragile family lines are if something as final as a gravestone doesn't match the few existing records. Since Rosina went by her husband's surname, Russo, when they married, but the cemetery recorded maiden surnames on gravestones, it must have been easy for names to be misspelled or incorrect, especially in a largely illiterate society. The maiden name would be lost over the years, and so, too, the ability to trace a woman's life.

"Jessica." Nonno jolted me from my thoughts. "We have found a sister." He pointed to a folio they had just pulled off the shelf. "Anna *Vienincasa*, and records of her brother, Antonio *Vienincasa*. There is a marriage certificate and a death certificate for Anna, but nothing else for Antonio."

"And Rosina's death certificate?"

"Sì." The woman pointed down to the handwritten pages. "Certificato di Morte. Vienincasa, Ro-seeenaaah."

She offered to type up copies of the records for a small fee. I asked if she could photocopy the pages instead, as the inky cursive with wide curls and sweeping letters could never be translated into Times New Roman, but she simply said, "No." While she typed up copies of the records, we waited outside near the church.

"Nonno, so that funeral card we found at your house of Anna, that *is* Rosina's sister?"

"It seems so. She was a few years younger than Rosina, her little sister, and she died before her."

I wonder if my children's children, and their children, will know that my sister was Melissa. That we spent Sunday afternoons together. That we looked alike even though we had different fathers. That, while our last names have never been the same, we were always closer than most siblings. How will that ever translate in records? And were Rosina and Anna close? How can I ever know that now?

Nonno walked over to the front step of the Comune. I kicked away the crunched cigarettes and tiny piles of grey ash and sat down next to him.

"Nonno, why was there nothing else for Rosina's brother, Antonio?"

"Since he was a very early emigrant, he didn't leave with the rest of us in the 1950s, so his records are who-knows-where. You know, he left just after the First World War and he went to America, not Canada. And he died there in a car accident, or something." Nonno shrugged. "His birth certificate"—he nodded toward the Comune—"said 1885."

Antonio died exactly one hundred years before I was born. "So, he was Rosina's younger brother. Do you think Rosina named her baby boy Emilo *Antonio* after him?"

"Probably." Nonno put his hand on my shoulder. "I'm going to go back in and pick up the copies."

I picked at the cracked paint on the railing beside me and thought about that sixth baby. He didn't even live until his first birthday. If his life was documented anywhere, the only records would be certificates of birth and death, and that space between, a dash separating dates on a grave marker, if he had one, would never reveal the impact of his life, or the way that Rosina loved him.

I looked up to see Nonno press open the Comune doors and step inside. I imagined two more red circles.

We walked through the narrow streets toward the house that Sisina's children had bought. We had heard that she now lived there. We stopped along the way to ask where the Casa di Sisina was, and everyone pointed down the hill.

We came to a tall, rectangular house with a huge garden full of bright pink rhododendrons open faced and soaking in the heat. When I pressed a petal between two fingers, the pink became a translucent red. There was a pile of marble cubes off to the side of the house and a wire coop with chickens pecking their beaks through the holes.

"Don't be disappointed if she can't remember anything," Nonno said as we waited at the front door.

"Geez. When you are Mr. Mario Ferrari, you sure are negative," I joked.

I heard the lock slide open, and then the wooden door opened a crack. Soon, Sisina stood before us, wearing a blue button-up dress with a lacy ivory slip poking out the bottom.

"Maaario? Mario!" Her voice was faint, but she seemed certain as she pulled him close and kissed his cheeks.

I glanced at Uncle, who threw his arms up.

"She remembers." I laughed.

Nonno held his arms around Sisina's shoulders as they walked through her hallway to the dining room. Uncle and I walked a few paces behind them, as he tried to translate for me.

"Uh . . . Calabrese, she speaks really true Calabrese. Something about . . . they were just talking about them, Mario and Rose. And Generoso. About the money that they all sent her from Canada to care for Rosina. Just yesterday Sisina and her daughter were talking about this."

"Yesterday?"

"I guess so!"

"All these years go by and they were talking about it yesterday?"

"Yeah, it seems so."

In the dining room, Nonno introduced me to Sisina. Her arms shook as she hugged me, then she held me an arm's length away, looked over my face, and nodded her head. Her hair was short and coarse, and much lighter than her dark grey eyebrows. Her glasses were perfect circles. Most of her teeth were missing. I could see some resemblance, though, between the first photo of Rosina and Sisina, now much older than Rosina had been in that photo.

She pulled out cookies and juice, and then sat down at a table draped in a thick white cloth.

"I can't understand a word," Uncle admitted to Nonno.

"Okay, you ask me the questions and I'll translate them into Calabrese. She does not speak that university-Italian stuff."

I had so many questions for Sisina, but it became apparent that I could only ask a few. They would be asked from me, to Uncle, to Nonno, and the answers filtered back the same way. It was faster for Nonno to translate from Italian to Calabrese than English to Calabrese. While they sorted out the questions and answers, Sisina just looked at me across the table.

"Okay, Jess. What do you want to know?" Uncle asked.

Everything.

I took a deep breath. "Okay. Once Rosina's husband, Giovanni, died, how did the house full of women, Rosina's four daughters, and her baby boy, Generoso, survive?"

When Nonno asked Sisina the question, she tilted her head back and closed her eyes. She nodded. And I waited for her words to reach me.

"They acted as men. The women worked the farm. Rosina worked night and day."

I imagined Rosina at dawn, up before anyone else, making bread and collecting chestnuts. I imagined her longing for Giovanni, a loss that not only left her lonely but forced her to work outside as a father and inside as a mother at a time when those roles had been so distinct.

"She was a strong woman," I said.

When my comment reached Sisina, she blinked slowly, and nodded. "Sì. Una donna forte."

"Why didn't Rosina remarry?" I asked. Sisina nudged a plate of cookies toward me and then pointed to my juice.

"It was important to keep land in the family. At this point, it was no longer about love. Only brothers could marry the widow. All of Giovanni's brothers were already married. You can't marry a stranger. And, she already had all of her children, so who would?" Sisina shrugged.

I noticed her gold wedding band in the folds of her finger. Her husband, Emilio Caupto, had died in 1963, just three years after Rosina moved in with them. Rosina must have understood Sisina's loss so well. I wondered if they had talked about it but couldn't bring myself to ask. It had been just the two women, Sisina and Rosina, in a tiny house somewhere in Grimaldi.

"What did Rosina feel when the rest of her family left for Canada?"

"You can't ask that," Nonno said.

"Why not?"

"How would she know?"

"Dad," Uncle explained, "they may have talked about it, just ask."

"Ah. Sì . . ." Sisina started. It took her a while to answer. "Rosina never showed any emotion. She was strong in every way. She was heartbroken once they were gone, but what could she do? She had a big heart. For anyone who stopped by, she'd mix up flour, water, and onion and cook them up. We lived just up the street, near the three fountains."

"Una donna forte," I said to Sisina and she nodded.

"Did Rosina move in with Sisina right after she moved out of the farmhouse in Maione?"

I imagined Rosina packing up her things, a few dresses, some dishes, and baskets for fruit. I imagined her waiting for the rest of the family to leave, one by one, until it was just Michelina and the youngest children left. It wouldn't be long until the house was empty.

"No, Jessica. She moved in with her daughter in Maione. Her daughter wasn't emigrating, but she fell ill and died. Her husband went to Sisina and said he couldn't handle being a caregiver. So they moved Rosina to Sisina's," Uncle said.

I imagined her packing up again. Her dresses folded over her arm.

"How many times can one person be moved?" I asked Uncle, looking through tears at Sisina. I had no way to explain my emotion to Sisina and I still had questions for her.

"Una donna forte, Jessica," he said and rested his hand on my arm. "What else would you like to know?"

"Was she clear in her mind?"

I wondered if she lay there at night and thought of all her losses: Giovanni, her daughters, her baby boy, her brother, her sister, her family to Canada. Or, maybe she forgot, one by one.

"Right until the end she was clear in her mind. She was against medication, even though Dr. Iachetta visited and tried to give her some. She spent the last years in bed. She couldn't even get out to use the washroom, but she knew everything and everyone. She didn't forget."

Sisina pulled out a stack of black-and-white photos. I saw a picture tucked underneath wedding photos sent from Canada. Nonno handed it to me. It was the largest version that I had ever seen, bigger than Nanni's eight by ten, and it had a once-white border, now curled up at the top and bottom. The image was almost the same: the wooden chair, the long black dress, the slight smile. The circles around her eyes. But everything was flipped and there was no background.

"Uncle, look. I don't understand," I said as I handed it to him.

"That's strange. It's the same photo but backwards. It must be a copy made from a slide."

Before I could examine the backwards photo, Nonno handed me a picture of a wedding party. "It's your nanni's brother, Giovanni. The one named after Rosina's husband. And look"—he pointed to a little girl off to the side—"that's your mother."

Mom had a big floppy bow on the top of her head, and she was wearing black Mary Janes with white socks pulled up to her knees.

"So, Giovanni sent this photo to his nanni Rosina. She had seen a picture of my mom, then?"

Uncle leaned in. "Yes. Sisina said these were Rosina's photos."

"Well! Is that it." Nonno made his question a statement. He grabbed a few cookies and swirled his cup of juice.

"If you don't mind, I'd just like to ask Sisina about Rosina's life as a midwife. There are so many stories about her delivering hundreds of babies. I always imagine her running through the night . . ."

"But, that's not really a question," Nonno said.

"We just want to hear stories, Dad. So, I'll try to ask," Uncle said.

Sisina looked confused, but then nodded and raised her eyebrows. She ran her hand over the twisted gold chain around her neck and then put her hands on the table. While I waited for her answer to reach me, I stared at the image of Rosina.

"Rosina delivered Sisina and most of the babies in the family. But she also delivered other people's babies. Sometime between 1950 and 1952 something happened."

"What happened?" I asked. Those were the years when the family started to leave for Canada. Generoso may have already gone.

"Well, you see," Nonno started.

I interrupted. "What did Sisina say, exactly?"

"Okay. She said Rosina was not a certified midwife. She just practised on her own. Everything was fine for all those years."

"And then?"

"Then, she went to deliver a baby, something went wrong. The mother. She bled. To death. She died. The baby girl, she's the one, the one that went to live with the nuns."

I felt my heart pounding and tried to look over at Nonno, to read his face, but he turned to Sisina.

Sisina, in a soft voice, said something while making a rolling gesture with her hand before she let it rest on the table.

"The villages kept it quiet. No one told on her. She could have been in serious trouble. Everyone kept the secret," Uncle translated.

"Sì," Nonno confirmed.

I leaned in to Uncle and whispered, "Is this baby girl the woman in Edmonton? The one Nanni knows?"

"Yes," Uncle answered.

"That's a true story, Jessica," Nonno said and reached for his glass.

QUATTRODICI

compass rose the centre of a compass that
displays the cardinal directions and orients
the traveller

We spent the next few days driving back to Rome. From the
back seat, I took in the bright Tyrrhenian Sea and coastal villages. We flicked through radio stations until we found songs
we knew, outdated American pop music, and listened until we
couldn't stand it anymore, and then we drove in silence except
when someone would poorly pronounce words on the signs or
interject with an anecdote from the trip. These short stories
would be among those tales told and retold about our going to
Italy, recited around the table during holiday meals.

The whiz of the wheels against the highway reminded me that we were on our way home. The souvenirs I had collected in Calabria were unlike those I'd found on other trips—no tiny flags, or specialty chocolate, no rocks or shells or trinkets. I spread out orange manila envelopes that contained birth and death certificates. The firm dates testified to the connections—lives that ran parallel, or came before, or came after—and the spans between these dates were the spaces for story. I didn't have any record of baby Emilio's life to show Nanni Rose, but I'd learned that Rosina and Giovanni's lives contained the loss of this seventeen-day-old boy. Emilio's story, the few weeks he existed, was perhaps somewhere between dates written in those handwritten folios, but maybe not. There may have been no records at all. I collected all of the pages and slid them into the backpack at my feet.

Sections of coastline slipped by the window; we crossed the border into the region of Campania. Nonno clapped his hands together. "Almost there now," he announced.

We were headed to the city of Salerno, where we had booked a room for the night. Nonno had seemed anxious to leave that morning, chatting about our schedule and the hours between Tonino's and the hotel as he lifted our bags into the trunk. He talked about our reservation while holding open my door, and that we could eat dinner once we'd arrived while buckling himself in and pointing to my seatbelt. Earlier on the trip, he had mentioned that this third visit would be his last to Calabria, but he told me I should go back one day, maybe build a little house and stay for a few months in the summer. We'd been in the car most of the day, and as the day sank into dusk, I wondered what Nonno was feeling.

"I can use your cellphone, right?" He was speaking to Uncle. "I want to tell your mother we left Calabria. I want to tell her when we get to the hotel."

"Yeah, Dad. Call her."

When we pulled into the hotel parking lot, I slid my backpack over my shoulders and then out of the car. Under the bright streetlights, the white lines scratched into the car—over the hood, the roof, the trunk, and across the doors—were visible. Uncle tried to buff one out with his finger. He shrugged and slammed the door shut.

"Andiamo," he sighed with less enthusiasm than the word demands. He nodded his head toward the hotel's white marble steps.

Before I even dropped my suitcase on the bed, Nonno was yelling into the receiver, "Eh-llo! Yep. Yep. We're here! Yep, Jessica is here beside me. Everybody is good. Yes, I left them a little money on my pillow, tucked it underneath 'cause I knew they wouldn't take it."

I decided to give him some privacy and went to the front desk to ask for a password for the Wi-Fi. Families were heading into the dining room, where I could hear the ching of glasses and the ting of utensils against plates and bowls.

"Buongiorno!"

"Buongiorno," I started.

"Hello. What do you require, miss?"

As the young man behind the desk slid a rectangle of paper into my hand and said, "You're welcome," I felt far from Calabria. Uncle walked through the lobby door and pointed at me. "Internet?"

"Sì!" I answered and wiggled the paper in the air.

"That's what I was coming for, too. Dov'è papà?"

"Nonno's on the phone in the room."

"Ha! Seems like we all felt a little disconnected. I need to check my work email, make a few calls, and find a place to make a reservation for tomorrow night."

As I made my way back to the room, kids ran by with rolled towels under their arms and goggles tight against their foreheads, and I felt like I had visited Maione and Altilia on another trip altogether.

"Back to reality, hey?" Uncle asked when he caught up.

"Yeah, making our way home," I answered and put my arm around his shoulder.

After dinner at the hotel restaurant, we slid our feet back to the room. Uncle reached into his suitcase and pulled out a bulbous jug of Francesca's limoncello.

"You realize you can't take that on the plane, right?"

"That's why we are having some now!" Uncle laughed and grabbed paper cups from the bathroom. After a few shots and flicking between news stations, they were both asleep. The low buzz of the old TV, rambling out sentences without stops, and the click of the air conditioner kept me awake. I didn't feel well—a little motion sickness from the day spent in the car. This nausea mixed with the weight of Sisina's words—Rosina's secret—and the sadness of leaving Calabria, a place I'd imagined myself so many times. I turned from my back to my belly and cried into my pillow.

I unzipped my suitcase and felt around for my laptop. Up until this point, I had only been using my laptop as a note keeper, a way to keep track of the family tree, because I didn't have access to the Internet. I wanted to send a message to my mom and Melissa until I was tired enough to fall asleep. After switching off the TV and bedside lamps, I shuffled across the cold marble floor to the bathroom. I didn't want to disturb them with the tapping of the keys.

I flicked on the fan and sat on the edge of the egg-white bathtub with a soft towel over my feet. I could see myself in the long-mirror: fuzzy curls, red eyes, sunburned face. With my laptop across my knees, I opened the screen and waited until it lit up. I entered the password from the front desk and waited a few seconds until I was connected. My stomach sank when he signed in. A tiny box in the bottom corner of the screen. His name in bold letters: Karl. I waited.

"Jess! I heard you're in Italy again."

I pushed the cursor into the tiny box. The line flashed there. I wanted to type something like, "Yeah, I'm here. I wish you were too," but I didn't. I typed and retyped a message until I finally pressed enter.

"Yeah, I'm here! Can you believe it? I swore I'd be back sooner. I miss you."

"You do?"

"Yeah. I do."

I held my hands against the smooth tub and waited for him to reply, but he didn't. He signed out or we lost connection. I closed the laptop and stood at the sink, remembering. When it all had finally ended, he had stood in the middle of the driveway. I said I was scared to have any firsts without him: we'd had them all together. He told me not to go. When I drove away, he didn't move from that spot. I know because I stared at him in the rear-view mirror until I reached the end of the block and had to turn off his street. Single moments can come to define an entire year. And years can be marked by befores and afters. The whirlwind trip to northern Italy was after the missed periods and before the breakup: the space between. I leaned my stomach against the counter and pressed my forehead against the mirror. I looked down at my body, my too skinny legs, my bony ankles, and my flat, hollowed-out belly.

I thought about *that* winter six years before. I imagined those bare-bone leafless trees in the front yard. Frozen limbs that could be easily snapped off, dropped into the snow. I remembered that it had hurt in my bones, my hip, my pelvis. I felt like they were rubbing against each other, grinding, even though I was still. I remember that I tried to sleep with my knees up against my stomach. I don't remember falling asleep. I had been concentrating on the perfect lines of the orange streetlight between the spaces of my venetian blinds.

I woke that night to a deep tug. Blood soaked through my sweatpants. It left a bright red bloom on my sheets. I shuffled to the bathroom, pressing my palms against the wall to feel my way there. I didn't want to see the blood in the light. Not yet.

I had pulled at the toilet paper and scrunched the long lines of paper in my hands. And then I saw it: a three-centimetre piece of pinkish tissue. I touched it with my finger. A bright line of blood trickled down my leg, and I scrubbed it off with a facecloth, though it remained on my skin, faint. And then I crouched down on the bathroom floor. I knew that my family would be awake soon. Alarm clocks would buzz. They'd fill mugs with coffee, slice up oranges, and pull the newspaper apart. My parents. My younger brother. I remember that everything was red.

I called Melissa.

"Hello?" Her voice was gritty with sleep.

"Melissa, I need to know how to wash out blood."

"Are you okay? What happened?"

"I lost a baby," I sobbed.

After high school graduation, after years of imagining a forever within the narrow frame of a teenaged life, Karl and I were suddenly thrust into the real world. This world included images we hadn't foreseen: blood droplets on the blue-tiled bathroom floor and a cotton ball bandaged into the crook of my arm.

We had outgrown the borders of Morinville years before we ever thought of applying for passports. We started planning our trip to Italy before I was pregnant and before I miscarried. We went anyway because we wanted to see some of the world together like we had planned, because we loved each other even if we sensed our little universe was coming to an end. We would lie in bed and imagine the spackled ceiling as stars that twirled in the glow of the muted TV, and we'd share wishes we knew would never leave the room.

❧   ❧   ❧

When I arrived home from Calabria, summer had drifted into fall. Frozen apples weighed down the branches of my parents' trees. Mom left the bruised ones in the grass for the birds to eat. The hedges around the yard were now red, rust, and yellow, but a rake could draw out the sweet smell of wet leaves ready to decompose.

I sat on the front steps, clutching a coffee between both hands. I thought of Tonino making me an espresso in the morning—a tiny cup with thick black liquid and brown foam and a tiny spoon to stir it with. Melissa and Mom sat in the patio furniture beside the steps, chatting about how cold it had become so fast. They waited to hear some stories about Italy.

And here she was too—Rosina. In new stories that belonged to the Old Country.

✿   ✿   ✿

She runs, alive with the night, shocked that it is happening so soon. Shadows spread across a worn path. The bright moon flashes between the trees and collides with the glassy light of the lantern in her hand as she goes. Her shadow rushes over the bony silhouettes of the trees on either side, lost to the darkness, to be lit up again in a stride. She had thought she would have at least another two weeks, maybe three, but when Maria tapped on the door just as she started to fall asleep, she knew.

"I'll come with you," she offered.

"No. No. You stay here. Rest. It's late."

She knows the ground well, even in the dark. She slows down around the spots where rotting roots have left holes and takes wider strides over a nettle patch; her legs are bare beneath her gown. There's a rush that comes with a night birth. A baby slips in to the world while neighbours are asleep in darkened houses and wayward husbands slumber somewhere under the stars. Nearby female relatives—aunts, sisters, mothers, and cousins—are awake and alert, ready to assist the midwife, to welcome new life. The exhausted mother pleads for rest in the seconds between the contractions that attack her body, force it to twist into a knot around her belly. She spits out the name Gesù! and belts hard *ahhhs* from her throat after she swallows strings of vomit.

When a flickering light in the window comes into view, Rosina runs faster, snapping the brittle grass as each foot smacks the ground. She feels dizzy; the tall trees look like deep green smudges, but the stars stay in place. She concentrates on planning her movements, imagines what could happen. What she will do if there is too much blood. If the water has not broken. If the cord is tangled. If the baby is crowning, or if its legs are pushing through first. *She's done this hundreds of times. Hundreds.*

She plunges her hands into a pail of water on the porch, splashing moonlit water onto the wooden steps. As she yanks open the door, heat from the fireplace flashes against her cheeks. In the corner, coffee boils on the stove, preparation for the long night ahead. The scent of dark beans and blood curls in the air. In haste she lets her bag slump off her shoulders and fall to the floor. The bag is teeming with herbal remedies, homebrews in corked jars. Puffy aloe leaves, cabbage, and containers of clover. Cloths, pressed and folded. Forceps, scissors, and sewing needles.

An oil lantern, hanging from a ceiling beam, spills pale yellow light across the floor. Women stare at her. They shuffle to make space and then look to her for direction. One says, "Come. Come. We've been waiting."

With her hands on the labouring woman's sticky thighs, her hip hard against the bed frame, Rosina presses the woman's legs apart and counts the number of beats between shudders. She instructs the others. You, hold her legs back—farther. And you, rub a damp cloth on her neck and lips to keep her cool. And someone, open the window and let the breeze in. Rosina's heart thumps deep in her chest and throbs behind her eyes, making it impossible to keep track. The others count; she trusts their heavy whispers. The woman has been pushing already and is soaked in sweat, and shaking. Her hands, balled into tight fists, are white, and her veins, bright purple lines, are thick with blood. Rosina takes the woman's hands into her own. Damp skin sticks to her palms. She uncurls the woman's fingers, reminds her to breathe, and with two fingers to the woman's wrist feels her pulse. Rosina brushes away the black curls, stuck to the woman's forehead and neck. She steps back for a moment and looks at the woman—two round breasts atop one round belly, swollen feet and fingers, puffy eyelids and lips, back arched, pushing everything she has forward. It might be too late. The bed sheets are stained with bright blood. The woman is weak, white. Some women speak to Mary. Some ask Mary to speak to God. *Let the surges stop. Let the baby come.*

After an entire night of labour—an entire house heaving together—a baby girl is born. Sunlight creeps in beneath the brown velvet curtains: a too bright, unwelcome rising. Daylight reveals lines of brown blood, tiny dry rivers, following the cracks of the floorboards. The women stare at the ground, following the rivers with their eyes, tracing the flow. The mother never cries out to Mary, Mother of God, because the mother never wakes to see the morning, and Rosina, the midwife, never tugs another life into the world. All of the women in the house agree to keep a secret. A secret that the whole village will bury in a hole in the ground in the hillside cemetery.

The baby rests in one of the women's arms and Rosina bends down to kiss her forehead. She shakes her head and whispers, "Mi dispiace." I'm sorry. It is a sorrow that will swell. She leaves her bag on the floor, her tools across the table, the sheets in a pile.

She makes her way through the woods and back to the farmhouse, where she will look up at the crucifix over her doorway and press her hand against her chest. By the time she gets home, her blood-covered hands will have soaked her white cotton apron, forming red circles that will never wash away.

It was yesterday
that I swam
across a winter-white field
until sheets tore off
and melted into sea
I saw you there
high up on a hill
snapping clothes pins
across the sky

Rosina
Giovanni

Terracina
Adelina
Maria
Palmira
Emilio
Antonio
Generoso
Michelina

Giovanni
Rose
DiFilippo
Vittorio
Maurizio
Maria
Mercandino

Lucianna
David

Melissa
Jason
Cory
Jessica
Joseph

SOURCES

I am greatly indebted to those writers who have created a body
of work that spans genres and speaks to the Italian Canadian
experience—from within Canadian borders and beyond. The
existence of the Association of Italian Canadian Writers (AICW)
testifies to the strong presence, and the network, of such writers
within the wider Canadian literary community. I am thankful for
this collection of voices from early accounts by Italian explorers
such as Giovanni Caboto, observing what is now Canada, to two
2012 publications on the internment of Italian Canadians during
the Second World War—made possible by a partnership between
the AICW, Guernica Editions, and *Accenti Magazine*. These voices
have informed and inspired.

For their direct influences, I owe thanks to the following historians, academics, essayists, poets, filmmakers, and creative writers for their works: Frank Anderson for *The Rum Runners* (Lone Pine, 1991); Stanislao Carbone for *The Streets Were Not Paved With Gold: A Social History of Italians in Winnipeg* (Manitoba Italian Heritage Committee, 1993); Adriana Davis for research and writing on the *Celebrating Alberta's Italian Community* web-site (albertasource.ca/abitalian); Caterina Edwards for *Finding Rosa: A Mother with Alzheimer's, a Daughter in Search of the Past* (Greystone, 2008); Francesco Loriggio for *Social Pluralism and Literary History: The Literature of the Italian Emigration* (Guernica, 1996); Antonino Mazza for many works, including *The Way I Remember It* (Guernica, 1992); Melania Mazzucco for *Vita: A Novel* (HarperCollins, 2006); tremendous thanks to Joseph Pivato for his body of work, especially his comprehensive essays, including "What Is Italian-Canadian Writing?" (athabascau.ca); Nino Ricci for *Lives of the Saints* (Cormorant Books, 1990) and *In a Glass House* (McClelland & Stewart, 1993); a great thanks to Franc Sturino for many works, including *Forging the Chain: Italian Migration to North America 1880–1930* (Multicultural History Society of Ontario, 1990); Vito Teti for *La Razza maledetta: Origini del pregiudizio antimeridionale* (Manifestolibri, 1993); and Nicola Zavaglia for the documentary *Barbed Wire and Mandolins* (National Film Board, 1997).

For other histories, I am especially thankful to the following authors: John A. Davis for the chapter "Italy 1769–1870: The Age of the Risorgimento" in *The Oxford Illustrated History of Italy* (Oxford University Press, 1997); Edward Marks for the article "Internationally Assisted Migration: ICEM Rounds Out Five Years of Resettlement" (*International Organization*, 1957); PBS for the documentary *The Sinking of the Andrea Doria* (2006); and Alice Trottier for *Faith and Tenacity: A History of Morinville* (Saint-Jean-Baptiste, 1991).

For their writing about midwifery, creative and historical, I am grateful to the following authors: J.H. Aveling for "On the Instruction, Examination, and Registration of Midwives" (*The British Medical Journal*, 1873), Ami McKay for *The Birth House* (Knopf Canada, 2006), Mariella Pandolfi for "Midwives, Godmothers, and Witches: Female Body and Identity in the Italian South" (*American Ethnologist*, 1993), Diane Vecchio for the comprehensive *Merchants, Midwifes, and Laboring Women* (University of Illinois Press, 2006), and Mariella Pandolfi for "Midwives, Godmothers, and Witches: Female Body and Identity in the Italian South" (*American Ethnologist*, 1993), among many, many others. I also thank Janice Kulyk Keefer for the inspiring memoir *Honey and Ashes: A Story of Family* (HarperCollins Publishers Ltd, 1998).

ACKNOWLEDGMENTS

I would like to thank my publisher, Ruth Linka, for believing in this book, and the fine, fine people at Brindle & Glass for making this project possible. I thank my editor for loving Rosina, and for coming with me, line by line, to Calabria and back—you are a gem, Linda Goyette.

For the striking cover photograph, thank you Henry Roxas. For the hand-drawn, beautiful map, the family tree, and the lettering on the cover, I thank you very much, Karl Sundquist.

I thank all of my University of Victoria workshop peers and instructors. Lynne Van Luven, without your engagement with my manuscript, this book would not exist. Thank you, David Leach, for asking important questions and telling me that I had to go to Calabria. Thank you, Lorna Crozier, for permitting me to be

poetic. Thank you, Melanie Siebert, and my MFA cohort: Amanda Jardine, Yasuko Thahn, Peter Boychuck, and Michael Nardone.

I am so grateful for the love and constant support of my parents: a heartfelt thank you, Mom and Dad, for encouraging me to write. Thank you to all my *famiglia* and my family-like friends from the top branches to the roots. I especially wish to thank my immediate family, Melissa, Jason, Cory, Joseph, Les, Robin, and Brandy, and dear friends Jenny and Karl for letting me write you into my stories. Thank you, Jim and Janet, for your readiness and willingness to support me.

Nanni and Nonno, I thank you for telling me stories.

A special thank you to Nonno for letting me stand on his doorstep. Thank you, Uncle Robert, for booking tickets to Calabria before you'd read a word.

I thank my Reid for reading my work, for supplying *that* word when it escapes me, for reminding me how to place commas, and, most of all, for always pushing me forward.

And of course, I thank Rosina, the midwife—who is always with me.

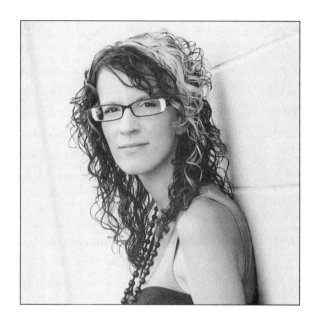

JESSICA KLUTHE's work has appeared in numerous literary publications including *The Malahat Review, The Writer's Block, Little Fiction*, and *Notebook Magazine*. Recently, Kluthe won the *Other Voices* creative non-fiction contest for an excerpt from *Rosina, the Midwife*. In 2011, she was shortlisted for the Alberta Writers' Guild James H. Gray award for the first chapter of this book. She received her MFA in writing from the University of Victoria. Kluthe is a writing instructor at Grant MacEwan University in Edmonton, Alberta, and is at work on a novel. Visit Jessica online at jessicakluthe.com and follow her on Twitter @jessicakluthe.